Determined to Get a *Life*

The Story Doesn't End with Dementia

KEN CRASSWELLER

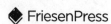 FriesenPress

One Printers Way
Altona, MB R0G 0B0
Canada

www.friesenpress.com

ISBN
978-1-03-916934-0 (Hardcover)
978-1-03-916933-3 (Paperback)
978-1-03-916935-7 (eBook)

1. BIOGRAPHY & AUTOBIOGRAPHY, PERSONAL MEMOIRS

Distributed to the trade by The Ingram Book Company

Acknowledgements

My thanks to God for Lesley now deceased, my wife and teammate, for some works she authored appearing within. To all with whom I conversed to hear their stories, To James Bay Care Home staff for understanding Lesley's Dementia. To journalist Ron Ellerton for his help, with appreciation to FriesenPress team for publication patience.

Foreword

The dead need to be where they go
The living go where they need to be.
—Anonymous

This book describes my wife's struggle with dementia and my determination to continue living on despite her death. One giant question visited me while I grieved: Did I want to go on living? Dementia, like a thief, took my life partner without allowing goodbyes. If the answer was yes, I did want to go on, how would I do that? Eventually the answer came. I found it by reconnecting with nature and with others, assuming both are necessarily linked.

During the time I cared for Lesley at home, a hospital social worker visited. One day she told me I looked a wreck and could no longer help Lesley by myself. I might even die before she did. The pain of hearing that became amplified when I read a newspaper obituary of a man who'd died two weeks after his wife's passing. Up until then, he enjoyed good health. Apparently, that was not uncommon. Still, that possibility shocked me, and made me want to help myself and others get a life after a loved one's death.

Preface

"There is a crack in everything
That's how the light gets in."
—Leonard Cohen

This effort consists of Book One and Two. The first is about Lesley and her journey through darkness. The second is about me confronting Lesley's dementia and death, arriving at a resolution to reconnect with life.

In this book, find details of incidents that prompted its appearance. Find also a collection of short stories set in a park, meet characters, and hear about their lives while riding a bus. Discover a litany of happenings all combined to support my decision to live on.

Meet Lesley, find out who she was and what happened to her while she suffered dementia.

In this book, I pose the question: What caused Lesley's dementia? Was it an accumulation of stressors? Did the turmoil in Lesley's brain create overwhelming static, short-circuiting messages? Or was it aging that caused her worn-out parts to shut down, and finally her brain? Or was it prescribed chemicals that "sent her round the bend"?

Finding it all so painfully hard to take, knowing Lesley had fought hard to survive, first at home, then in care centres, I eventually, reluctantly, made choices others like me may benefit from reading about what I learned and ultimately did.

I will try offering answers to these questions:

- When Lesley was going through hell, what did I do?
- How did I feel about what was happening to Lesley throughout her journey and at the end?
- Given two choices, fold or play, what did I decide to do after tapping helpful resources, and what did I conclude would be the best path to closure? I will detail how I did this, by looking neither to the past with regret, nor to the future with apprehension. But by living in the present I got a life after Lesley's death.
- How did I do that? Answer: by reconnecting with nature and with others, feeling both together a must for a bereaved person to recover and live on.

After Lesley's death I turned to recalling two experiences: the first walking around a park parameter, talking to people along the way and fantasizing about waterfowl, connecting with nature. The second , conversing with individuals listening to their personal stories while out of our natural element, in a confined space —a bus.

Another experiential message of this book, is enhanced by voices of great inspirational minds.

When someone special to you dies, the "give up" attitude thrives. You forget the essential ingredient of life still exists. Namely : Visualize, connecting with nature and others, it can be likened to the sacrament of sharing bread and wine, bread representing gifts of nature, wine representing human life.

The death of a loved one nullifies the declaration "The two now are one." What happens when we are no longer two, but once again, only one? Nature, hand in hand with other people, restores the will to live on, which is in essence the message of this book.

What might that look like for you? Would it be daily sitting in a park with nature and talking to people? For me, this was communing, engaging in the lives of others to reconnect to my energy source, the place where death had left a space, filling it instead with life? One is reminded of a pottery studio, in which you kneaded clay (that's the person) and a flux (that's nature) to create a beautiful new glazed work of art.

But a problem can surface if a bereaved person had gained identity, meaning, and purpose from only the deceased. Inherent in this book's content is the question:

Could the surviving member, solo, or become a defeatist, declaring, "I'm nothing without you"?

It's possible, and practical, to continue remembering, celebrating, thankful for one's partner's life without feeling guilty as the one still alive and kicking. Could it be helpful to vow to carry on honouring what the deceased represented and still get a life?

In summary, the formula for dealing with death of a person once close and intimate is, simply put: connecting with nature + people = peace of mind and a way to live on!

It worked for me. Would it work for you or another? It should. Why? Because we need nature and nature needs us, nature to nurture the mind, and humans to mind it.

Table of Contents

BOOK ONE

"Do not go gentle into that good night,
Old age should burn and rave at close of day;
Rage, rage against the dying of the light."
—Dylan Thomas

Chapter 1: Before Deep Dementia

When I think of Lesley, I hear "Spirit, Spirit of Gentleness" by John K. Manley, and Roger Whittaker's song "The Last Farewell."

Lesley read prolifically, did crosswords, sang in a choir, lead worship services, practised TaiChi, conversed with church and CGIT girls group leaders friends, and wrote (having journalist's skills). She, a people person with leadership skills brought positive responses from all whose lives she touched.

Then something happened. Lesley's vibrancy and confidence took a turn for the worse. It became evident one day when she gazed at a storm-at-sea picture I'd painted and softly said, "That's the way I feel inside."

Many weeks passed with Lesley showing fear, feeling

she was descending into a dark place. Her doctor referred her to the local hospital gerontologist for assessment. Many visits followed.

At first, I'd often found Lesley—long past midnight—asleep on the couch with a book open in her hands, as if still reading. I'd help her to bed, and then I began taking on more of the household chores and morning and bedtime routines. Lesley accepted my role, leaving me with the understanding that I would from then on be her caregiver in every way.

Lesley seemed to realize her limitations and often said, while watching me fumble around, doing what she once did so capably, "You shouldn't have to do that."

Chapter 2: Lesley's Journey

The Bird at the Window

"Winter had come to the prairies. The storm pelted the window with sleet and snow as the man settled to read before crackling logs in his fireplace. Soon a *thud, thud* on his windowpane brought him back to think of the night outside. A near-frozen, panic-stricken bird darted desperately, crashing into the window time and time again. The man opened the door to let the bird come into his warm home. But the wild bird could not understand, and would not fly in.

Leaving his warm house, the man opened his door and lit a small heater hoping to lure the bird inside. Still, it refused to come in. Really frustrated, the man called out, "Oh, if only I could be a bird for one minute so I could show you what I've been trying to tell you! Anon

What Was Happening to Lesley?

Disturbed by what I saw happening to Lesley, I began trying to cope with the gradual loss of who she once was. Her doctor found evidence of her brain dying a little at a time. I saw Lesley regressing gradually, passing through different life stages, ultimately on a journey back to infancy.

Lesley's downward slide over many months caused us to relocate to different living arrangements, to accommodate regrettable changes. The moves were stressful to my dismay; Lesley found different ways of expressing her frustration,

Lady Simcoe Apartment:
"There is Something Very Wrong With Me!"

Lesley looked distressed, and often asked me, "What is happening to me?" We again visited her doctor, who felt she was sinking into depression. The doctor prescribed an anti-depressant. She took it for a while, with adverse results. Lesley then consulted the internet and read, "This should not be given to anyone over age sixty-five." Finding that disturbing, she got a different anti-depressant.

In the weeks and months that followed, Lesley lost interest in crosswords. Once an avid reader, she found she kept reading the same page over and over, no longer able to advance along in any book. One day she asked me again,

"What is happening to me?" I had no feeling sad. Thereafter, she stopped reading.

Days passed. Often Lesley said fearfully, "I feel strange pressure on my head, like the tightening of an elastic band." A referral by her doctor to the hospital gerontologist led to many physical and exploratory tests resulting in no definitive answers or cure. Lesley continued to visit the hospital specialist, who monitored her memory loss and deterioration with tests, never mentioning dementia to Lesley.

A pharmacologist working with the hospital specialist monitored the anti-depression dosages. Days passed, with Lesley growing more fearful of me yet furious when I left her alone while I worked out at the YMCA. Yet while shopping for groceries with me, she often wandered off getting lost among the shelves. I started to feel uncomfortable having to tell her what to do, when and how. Before dementia, strong-willed, like me, she wouldn't stand for that. After dementia surfaced, she became disturbingly compliant.

Ross Place: "Do You Know Where Lesley Is?"

Lesley and I decided to move from Lady Simcoe, where we had lived for thirteen years to Ross Place, an independent living arrangement. Our move was in step with Lesley's decline. Neither she nor I were able to settle in, unfamiliar with the luxury and the perceived lack of friendliness.

Lesley wandered sometimes from our apartment. Once, there was a knock on our door:

"Do you know where Lesley is?"

"Why, yes," I said. "She is with me."

It was not so. While I'd been watching TV, Lesley had stepped out. I found her in the basement staff room, hugging a teddy bear.

I recalled, back at Lady Simcoe Lesley left without telling me, She had found her way, to a cafe "to meet her friends," only later lost coming home. Another knock on the door.

Rose Manor: "Leave Me Alone, I'm Talking to My Friend"

With Lesley showing no interest in what Ross Place offered, Rose Manor became our new home. Lesley showed no excitement or keen interest in our walks together, church, or anything once important to her. It seemed her world was shutting down, less available to her.

Then She she began to lose interest in food, leaving our assigned table to "visit her friends" at another table. Often on our way back to our apartment, Lesley became angry with me for interrupting her conversations. I felt she saw me as the "devil incarnate."

One episode followed another till our gerontologist's social worker intervened. She convinced me again I was a wreck, and, as a caregiver, at my wits end. With Lesley obviously hurting and I inadequate, both of us deteriorating, I arranged a placement in Oak Bay Lodge, a place offering care to dementia patients.

Oak Bay Lodge:
"I Know What You Are Doing"

We drove to the door of the new place. I stepped out of the car. When I moved toward the Lodge door, Lesley shouted, "I know what you are doing!" That just about broke my heart.

Following hugs, I stayed with Lesley while staff helped her settle in her room, which she was to share with another lady.

Weeks followed. I visited Lesley, soon finding that room didn't work for her. She didn't seem comfortable with strangers. What followed was an instant, escorted rush down a hall into another part of the facility where Lesley was given her own room. Why had the caregiver insisted on whisking my wife down the hall, with me running behind to keep up? Was it for fear that Lesley would balk at the idea and cause a fuss? I never got an answer.

More weeks passed with the promise that after two months following this first obligatory placement, she and I then would have the power to find Lesley more suitable accommodation elsewhere. During that waiting time, Lesley suffered a severe arm fracture from a fall while walking the halls at Oak Bay Lodge. It requiring many hospital visits.

James Bay Care Home

I found a place for Lesley in James Bay Care Home, and an apartment for me in Lady Simcoe—where Lesley and I had enjoyed rental occupancy for thirteen years. That made visiting much easier, for I lived minutes away down the street from Lesley.

I still remember when we first arrived at the door of her new home, Lesley was greeted warmly, and to the pleasant surprise of the greeter, she sweetly smiled, and blew the greeter a kiss.

Revealing Moments

Before and after Lesley's arrival in her new home, she struggled to construct sentences, resulting in gibberish. But sometimes she did surprisingly find words to succeed in sharing her needs or feelings. It was then I still saw glimpses of Lesley rising from the dark depths of her dementia.

*

The hall was long, Lesley tightly grasped my hand, her finger nails digging deep. She tugged, urging me on. Her eyes pleaded for understanding, repeating "I'm only a kid, you know!" sought patience! And if it was not my hand to grasp along the way, another would do. Sometimes this other reluctant resident looked bewildered and fearful.

*

"You always get your own way!" Lesley sometimes blurted out when I had her join me for walks. Often when she walked with me, outbursts followed. Growing angry, she would charge ahead, not looking back. When I'd caught up, sometimes stopping ,she'd quietly, say "I'm sorry."

*

Sometimes in the care home garden or on walks, I would point out different flowers as we went along. Lesley would echo my word: "Pretties."

*

Other times, when visiting Lesley she'd approach me looking very fearful saying, "They're trying to kill me!" Was it medication causing her paranoid? Perhaps Lesley was reacting to side effects—or revealing a deep sense of insecurity?

*

Lesley abhorred baths, always making a fearful fuss She often grew angry too when helped to dress or undress, crying, "No! No!"

I felt so sad when dementia took away Lesley's sense of dignity, and pride of person.

*

For some months, Lesley carried around dolls and stuffies, seemingly showing affection for them. But when one visitor tried praising her for how she cared for her baby, she'd responded indignantly, saying, "It's a doll!"

Searching for an explanation to share with staff and visitors, I said Lesley once had a miscarriage years ago: Perhaps flashback memory of that loss?

Visiting

The Covid pandemic and subsequent care home lockdown stopped me from visiting Lesley for three months. On the first visit back, she said, " You finally found me." evoking my tears,

Most of my visits with Lesley before Covid ended with Lesley growing angry. This amplified whenever I started to leave. She'd shout choice words including "bugger" adamantly insisting I must stay with her. The only way I could get away was if a care worker distracted her. To my relief, that worked, with Lesley responding to encouraging similes, touching and hugs.

During "Covid, Lock Down, " Lesley and I could have talked on the phone while I stood outdoors seeing Lesley through a window, or could shout over the fenced-off barrier while Lesley sat in the garden. None of those options would work because of Lesley's hearing, seeing, and processing limitations. Lesley read lips so masks muffled voice contact even more.

Over time she became less concerned about her appearance and problems communicating. Her caregivers tried their best with her partial denture. d keeping hearing aids in her ears. Impossible! Essential items disappeared. Others appeared. "Where is Lesley's walker? Someone else has it? It's got to be somewhere!" Lesley would shrug her shoulder, showing no interest or concern when I, in a flap began the hunt for the missing as often happened.

Eventually, realizing my concerns became a nuisance to the caregivers, I backed off nagging, recognizing caregivers, available 24/7 demonstrated real ethnic respect and empathy for the elderly.

I felt Lesley's world slowly closing in on her and accepted that my concerns were not hers, nor those of her practical, very devoted caregivers.

Still, despite dementia's darkness, I marvelled at Lesley's strong will, her "onward and upward" inner strength and spirit, which drove her on. That somehow served her well in that topsy-turvy, off-kilter, locked, second-floor ward. Lesley's caregivers said, "She was a very busy person"; She determined to fight on, refusing to give up or give in charging up and down the hall, stopping briefly to crane her neck to peer into rooms, try exit doors, and cling to the hand of anyone passing by, not letting go.

More than once touching moments happened. One day Lesley stopped in flight, reached through one restrained resident's half-open door, to gently touch a lost soul's outstretched hand. Lesley's kind, gentle act reminded me of how, over the years, she had comforted so many. It was a brief moment captured from the past. Compassion still existed within her.

She would often stop pacing the hall, walk into the small nursing station space, and peer at a staff member without speaking posing the question, "Why?"

"Where is Lesley?" was a question I often asked when visiting. I'd find her leaning over a sink, busy scrubbing a piece of cloth. I'd take her by the hand back to her room, sit a bit. Soon she'd, grasp my hand, yank me up, point to the door then away we'd go up and down the hall again.

By contrast, Grace, an empathetic whirlwind visitor, would take Lesley by the hand, engendering fun, swinging arms and dancing joyfully up and down—to Lesley's delight.

I often felt helpless leaving after a visit, I'd sometimes hear Lesley screaming as caregivers helped attend to her other demeaning needs.

I'd try to rest easy, hearing a caregiver shout assurance, "It's okay, Lesley isn't being hurt."

"Where is Lesley?" She wasn't sleeping in a chair or pacing the floor. She is asleep in another resident's room, often flaked out when out of steam from hall walking.

Lesley stayed awake throughout most nights, sitting sleeping through the day when not doing her hall rounds. Staff tried ways she could sleep through the nights by moving her bed outside the nursing station window, tried sitting beside her till she slept. Nothing seemed to work.

When visiting, I'd lead her often out into the garden, but after a brief walk around, pointing out flowers or other features, with her staying silent, she would head back to the door, having had enough. Inside I'd point out the aquarium's fish. No response. I wondered, though, why whenever a caregiver would plunk a sunhat on her head, she'd smile.

We went for walks. sat eating ice cream. No matter what I pointed out or talked about, she spoke gibberish as always.

I once spoke to Lesley in a dream; she said she used gibberish because she wanted to stay safe in the nursing home, thinking if she didn't she'd not qualify to be there, forced to leave as a normal person. Could that be true?

During Covid Lockdown, I sent Lesley cards, photos, and chocolate bars, asking a caregiver to sit with Lesley and share the cards' messages.

But that was no substitute for the show of affection demonstrated before Covid when Lesley and I greeted each other, I with open arms, Lesley snuggling in close with hugs evoking "awwws" from pleased staff,

I decorated Lesley's room walls with pictures, family

photos and other memorabilia, including her first class best flower award. Sometimes she'd struggle to make sense of what was there, her gaze strained and puzzled. In contrast, remembering walks down the hall at Oak Bay Care home, Lesley would look at a wall in passing, point to the word Lesley, smile, and say, "That's me." I felt sad and exhausted for her. She often appeared lost and distant; then sometimes surprisingly, out of the dark a spark of recognition would appear in her eyes.

I marvelled at her inner spirit, or the last vestige of it, which drove her onward, despite fear and the constant exhausting effort, moment by moment, to reorient her to the space surrounding her. It hurt so much watching her look for a door to leave by after a short visit with me, to again head out down the hall on a quest for something unknown. Then I wistfully remembered the way it once was for Lesley in the first few words of the hymn, Spirit of Gentleness *by* James Manley (1975). It was in keeping with Lesley's indomitable spirit flowing through Dementia's wilderness.

Before, thinking years back lost but not forgotten glowed her spirit enhanced by her dear friend-like sister Marjo's annual visits and walks shored up by who Lesley once was in such cherished relationships.

Yet, I felt so distraught when cherished friends Carol and Tom made a trip especially to visit Lesley. It went badly. We sat together outsider the bed and breakfast.

Lesley and Carol had for years been very close, sharing leadership of a Taber church girls' group called Canadian Girls in Training,("CGIT") Lesley called Carol her daughter; Carol called Lesley her "CGIT" mom. Our expectation of a good visit quickly deteriorated into Lesley shouting, cursing, and tugging my hand to get away from our friends. Dumbfounded by Lesley's outburst, I reluctantly, with apology, led Lesley down the street, back to the care home. The only way I could get my head around what had happened was to accept that fear of the unfamiliar outdoor space had triggered her outburst. She was only at her best in small familiar spaces and within about seven feet of another person. She just wanted to get back to where she felt safe, surrounded by familiar caregivers.

That also often happened when I walked with Lesley around the James Bay community.

It would become evident that Lesley felt uneasy, beyond her comfort zone, namely, the James Bay Care Centre, her home.

Accepting Reality

A formidable task lay ahead for Lesley and me ended by accepting reality. I still often fussed around, getting in the way, a nuisance to the caregivers, no doubt, by making known my concerns, despite what they were doing in Lesley's best interest. I questioned her dosage of antidepressants. Was that the cause of her fears and outbursts?

I shared my concern as a question: Was it dementia or drugs that triggered her to say, "They are trying to kill me," the few words that broke through her usual incoherent gibberish? I became anxious over the doctor's dosage instructions: "Dosage as need be." I interpreted that as, "Use these drugs to control Lesley," or, "Snow her," which was a term I think I heard mentioned.

I felt myself gradually losing contact with Lesley, especially when she showed symptoms of increased paranoia.

It hurt seeing her rapidly losing weight; it came to a point where she had no interest in eating at all. She wouldn't enter the dining room, preferring to eat from a tray. Staff assured me they gave her Boost, or Ensure (nutritious substitutes,) and ice cream, something she enjoyed. Despite staff's attention to food for Lesley, she'd often just grab a cheese sandwich and, shuffle down the hall, sometime absently swinging it about. Nevertheless, I could see her wasting away.

Amid this painful witnessing Lesley's struggle to stay sane, safe, and moving, I sometimes heard the voice of one angry resident shout, "She's dying, you know!" Fortunately, Lesley, without her hearing aids, probably never heard it.

There were touching moments, though. One day when I arrived for a visit after lockdown, I saw Lesley, like an elegant lady sipping tea from a China cup held for her by a young caregiver.

Another time, after a visit, in the downstairs room designated for visiting during Covid, Lesley got up, leaving me sitting. She found a door, got away from the nearby caregiver, rushed down an office hallway, and entered a room. Two caregivers took her by the arms and gently led her to the elevator to the second dementia ward. She accepted her escorts like an important lady, allowing the honour of leading her back to the safety of her room.

The End

Then came the sad day when I was called in to be with Lesley at her bedside during the hours of her impending death. The doctor sat; his assistant stood by. I had decided, no heroics, Lesley would not go to hospital and be invaded by tubes and respiratory aids. Rather, her irregular breathing would gradually stop. I asked, and the doctor agreed, to have the oxygen that fed through her nostrils removed. She would be kept comfortable, free of excruciating pain, and would die with dignity, in keeping with her approach to life.

Lesley breathed her last during the brief time I spent at home The caregiver called me back to Lesley's bedside. Her body died at 7:00 p.m. in the James Bay Care Home on November 20, 2020 .in the same month and year that her twin, Keith died in Winnipeg.

Meeting Lesley While Flower Shopping (a dream)

I met with a flower shop salesperson who had known Lesley. I told her I'd recently seen a lady walking around the store, seemingly in a daze, picking up armfuls of flowers. Someone said the person looked like Lesley. The salesperson approached the lady. No, that wasn't Lesley, but Lesley often did wander about, looking lost, when I came shopping. The salesperson told me what happened. She had gently taken the flowers from the lady, who hadn't made a fuss.

Then the salesperson was approached by Lesley, who came up to her and smiled so beautifully, so sweetly. The salesperson gave Lesley some bits and pieces of leftover sales orders. They were mostly in little plastic pots. I was nowhere in sight, and the salesperson found in Lesley's coat pocket the slip of paper with the care home telephone number and address. On more than one occasion in the past, Lesley had wandered off and was found sitting on the curb, waiting for me The salesperson phoned the care home this time, to tell a nurse what had happened, and to let her know store staff would see that Lesley and her flowers got back home safely. There was silence on the other end of the line. Then the care home nurse softly said, "Lesley died in November, over a year ago."

The saleslady gasped, phoned me. She explained about meeting Lesley, and giving her the flowers.

After a long pause, I said, "That's okay. Things like this happen often in my dreams I understand and believe. I'll take the flowers you gave her to my home. There I will find room for them as I have for memorials of many moments and dreams of Lesley's presence Thank you!"

"There is a crack in everything that God has made."
—Benjamin Blood

What I Felt and How I Reacted to Lesley's Many Moments of Struggle

When I try to come to terms with my deep loss, I hear Lesley's words and remember how I felt during those moments. Each time I stepped into and out of a bewildering space and onto the next.

I felt for her, as no doubt the caregivers in the nursing home must have felt, watching her bravely each moment trying to reorient where she was, not able to rely on her memory. I felt for her carrying those painful pictures and feelings with me in between my visits and throughout the years since her death.

BOOK TWO

This is my account of one person, no doubt among many, who dealt with the death of a loved one who succumbed to dementia, and how I, among the bereaved, decided to live on a little more to enjoy a purposeful life, as Lesley had.

Introduction

In Book One I gave a picture of Lesley's struggle on her journey through dementia. I shared what I saw and felt, keeping in mind the fact that others, loved ones and friends of a dementia sufferer, also confront the same feelings and questions needing resolution.

Here, in Book Two, I keep in mind the fact that often a bereaved spouse dies within weeks of the death of his/her loved one, and often for no medical reason. I tell why and how I came to terms with Lesley's death, deciding to live on by turning to my resources, thinking others may decide to do the same. How did I do it? By reconnecting with people and nature walking, making stops along the way in a journey around Spirit Lake Park.

Chapter 3: How I Responded to Lesley's Death

In moving deeper into the darkness and despair of dementia, I believe many detailed experiences along Lesley's painful journey were lost. But the fear and anxiety remained to nag and haunt her as she regressed, until finally shouting out in frustration and anger, blasting, "I'm only a kid, you know!"

And what about that journey into darkness, and finally death?

I have a hunch the trauma of the war years pushed deep, lying subliminal in Lesley's sub-conscious, remaining there while she intensely engaged in motherhood, professional and volunteer endeavours. The sights and noisy fearful sounds of and despair surfaced only when Lesley retired.

The question was this: Did post-traumatic illness make

Lesley's dementia journey even worse than I perceived it to be?

I think back to what Lesley did and said and what my response was, how I felt at first trying to get in touch with her's and my feelings. I would often say when trying to reach her, "Remember when you told me about___?" I saw by her painful facial expressions her struggling to find meaning and sense of it all. Repeatedly during my visits I would forget that Lesley was no longer able to share with me our cherished connections that had enhanced our marriage. That hurt. For Lesley, that nurturing understanding had sunk into the darkness of dementia, and for me it had sunk into the darkness of despair. Loss left me with choices and decisions about whom or where to turn to for inner peace seeking a conviction to go on living. What I did with the leftovers of my experiences equipped me to live on.

Death and Dying, Kubler-Ross and Colleagues

I sought resources on how I could come to terms with deep loss. I found it partially in views of death and dying (*Good Therapy Blog* on the internet), by revisiting Kübler-Ross's Five Stages of Dying model. I applied it not only to my understanding of the needs of a dying person, but to my understanding of my own grief.

Kübler-Ross (KR) proposed one's journey to come to terms with death included these stages, in order: Denial,

Anger, Bargaining, Depression, and finally, Acceptance.

But I understood other models spelled out different views. Two suggested KR's inadequate and offered, instead, different models. One suggested "Reorganization, Healing and Renewal of a Sense of Identity." The other offered four basic steps: "Accepting the Reality of Loss, Experiencing Pain and Grief, Adjusting to the Environment, and finally, Redirecting Emotional Energy." Still a last voice, of psychologist Warden's, in my opinion, tossed out KR's sequential "Five Stages of Dying" one needs to go through and offered instead: "The ability to give and receive, to lean into and embrace the pain of loss while focusing on compassion and self-care. That I assume would include telling the story of the loss, exploring thoughts and feelings accompanying the story. (Bereavement 2011)

This last view of death and dying appealed to me more than the others. However, partially dissatisfied with that approach, I chose instead to incorporate my feelings, thinking, and actions by reconnecting with life through contact with nature and others, including their stories.

Beginning to embrace the decision to live on, I chose that way to step out of my grieving, letting go to reconnect with people, realizing we are a part of every person whom we've met, every person that has touched our lives.

Lesley often still enters my dreams and thoughts, evoking choking tears. What follows here is my attempt to do closer.

Chapter 4: Contributors to Lesley's Dementia?

After one painful visit with Lesley, I sat at home wistfully staring into space, remembering her sharing vivid flashbacks in a story that she wrote long before suffering dementia,

Over our sixty years married Lesley often reluctantly shared with me experiences of her's and Keith's childhood years. She and her brother would recall events of the war that occupied most of their childhood years. They laughed a lot, but also remembered fear.

They were eight years old by September 1939, light hearted, athletic youngsters whose parents believed their "kids" still had a future, sparked by hopes and dreams like those thousands of others yet unaware of that permanent lost carefree childhood,

In 2004, Lesley wrote of that lost childhood.

Just Gas Mask Kids

The ack-ack guns on the seafront boomed again, a reminder of September 3rd, 1939, when I and a bunch of my friends walked home from school.

"Hey kids, you know what? This afternoon at three o'clock, a whistle will blow and then the sirens, and then the bombs will start to drop on us." My stomach lurched, while glancing at my know-it all friend.

Keith, my twin brother and I scurried home. I knew a war was coming, but not so soon, not like that. My brother grinned at me, and I knew I had more time. The first siren came while I was leaning against the tall pole upon which it was fastened, trying to tighten the foot clamp on my roller skates. With first wail of the beast, I broke the record for an eight-year-old scampering home to safety, but not without first falling over.

Reassured it was only a test, both Keith and I took to the outdoors, as we usually did, scanning the skies for aircrafts, while hoping not to see any.

For six years we lived a life filled with snippets of conversation gleaned from eavesdropping on the many grown-ups of our large family. Living in the southeast corner of England, we were to have firsthand encounters of a horrible kind.

Gas masks—how we loathed us! I said I was always

afraid there was gas lurking in the mask and it would come out if I breathed too deeply. We carried everywhere—to school and Sunday school and while running around vulnerable. The masks were housed in square cardboard boxes, which quickly became makeshift footballs, often with masks inside.

Sometimes when we sat in our school air raid shelter, the principle would order the class to "don masks." We desperately tried to cheat by sticking our fingers inside the masks so we could breathe real air. We usually got caught in the act as teachers came to make sure the masks fit snugly.

The school shelters were fun at first, Our class raced in orderly lines from the school and down the shelter steps to fling ourselves onto the hard benches. Teachers handed out milk and cookies if we were there long enough. But they soon got around to ordering our students to take our books with us as we ran. The kids stalled bringing books, but then often forgot paper or pencils. The lights were very dim and so we were in our rights, claiming, "Please, sir, we can't see the words."

Then we would sing, trying to drown out the sound of planes and gunfire.

Usually after the sirens sounded the "all clear," we were allowed to run home.

Keith and I would usually loiter along, eagerly searching the sky for airplane dog fights until an air raid warden shooed us off, saying, "You kids run along home. You should not be out here."

We made plans to fight the enemy. Keith knew how to make Molotov cocktails, he told me . We planned to make some, climb a tree and hurl the bomb at any approaching enemy. Never mind we couldn't buy petrol and had no empty bottles with which to make the bombs, nor the fact that, as Keith distinctly put it, "You know, if we saw enemy soldiers, we wouldn't climb trees, we would run like hell."

He was nine years old by then, and full of wisdom!

*

Uncle Charlie was a hero, He was a soldier and was also married to my mom's oldest sister, Auntie Min .She lived across the road from us in our grandmother's house.

Uncle Charlie went overseas early in the war. Keith and I heard lots of anxious talk by eavesdropping around our aunts and uncles over at Gran's house.

Finally, the news of Dunkirk was on the radio and in the newspapers—and Uncle Charlie came home, rescued by some brave soul.

Skulking around, Keith and I picked up snippets of Uncle Charlie's exploits. The one fascinated us the most had us running to our corner grocery and regaling the owner with tales of how our uncle and some other soldiers were actually rounding up prisoners when the order to retreat and evacuate came through. What to do with the prisoners? One of Charlie's sidekicks turned on his prisoner with his bayonet fixed, said Charlie, and he begged for mercy. But his pal said, "Mercy, you? I'll give mercy," and he bayoneted the prisoner.

The store owner must have blanched at this filth coming from the lips of two nine-year-olds, although the only comment I remembered was, "Oh, really?"

Anyway, the twins' obvious eavesdropping was severely curtailed, making the kids realize our tale-bearing had been brought to our elders' attention.

Uncle Charlie was later sent to Italy, where he was wounded and kept as a prisoner in an Italian hospital before being shipped off to a POW camp.

He wasn't the only one in the family to be evacuated from any place. As the pace of the war increased, the government ordered the evacuation of children from coastal areas. I recalled some families sent our children to North America and didn't see us again until the war ended in 1945. My mom and aunties conferred and decided us kids would not go overseas, only inland.

So one day, we twins were sent trudging along to the railway station with our gas masks, name tags on our lapels, and our bag lunches. Our schoolteachers and principal were with us. All the moms were crying, which didn't help ease the pain of parting. Our mom gave Keith last instructions: "You make sure you two stay together." I remembered it was a long trip. Our teachers didn't say much to us on the train.

We didn't even stop us from eating our lunches too early. I remembered one teacher slowly eating a great big bag of gooseberries. She didn't share. I hoped the teacher would have a stomach-ache.

We reached our destination, were taken to a big hall with long tables, and fed by a bunch of volunteers. We were put into groups, led by more volunteers with lists of names and addresses. Our sister and cousin, four years older, went with another group. Keith and I were put in a group of seven or eight kids, and we went trudging up and down the streets. The people on the list were locals who'd offered to take one or two evacuees, and we were being delivered—one kid here, two more there. Keith clutched my hand as though our mom's eyes were on him.

Problems arose when we reached one house. The lady who came to the door looked us over and said, "I'll take the boy." Keith's hand tightened as he said, for the first time of several times, "My mom said we have to stay together." After considerable bickering, the lady finally relented, said I'd take two instead of one. I remembered I didn't like the lady, and the lady didn't like me, so we were soon even. The lady had two girls around ten, so they welcomed having Keith around. But I thought the girls didn't like me much. They were probably afraid they would have to babysit us or something.

As evacuees we shared a school with the local kids, which meant we went to school half days. Things brightened when all the moms were allowed to visit, and all the kids got to show us off to the people boarding us.

Finally, when the bombing on the coast and London got the worst, most women were evacuated inland, so we got to see more of our mom. In a short time, our mom and aunties got together and decided Hitler wasn't going to chase us out of our homes. So we charged back to our mom's home in Seaford with us kids in tow. So many other parents reclaimed their kids and homes that the authorities couldn't stop them.

Shortly after we returned, we learned of the "terror of the night." Dimly awake, aware only of our father's outstretched arms and hearing nothing but the mad, wailing shriek that had never left our minds, we leaped upwards to be caught in the arms and hustled to the air raid shelter.. In the morning our terror was somewhat relieved when we discovered that our school had been bombed. Our fun didn't last long; the arrangement was made for classes to happen in the high school.

Another raid happened before the air raid siren sounded. The family was sitting near our fireplace when suddenly there was a huge whoosh, and then a sort of blackness. I realized I was on my hands and knees in the corner of the room, and all the lights were out. Mom was hollering because the windows were broken. I didn't know where Keith was. I didn't remember when I had been blown out of her chair. I just was!

I did remember how, sometime in the terror, my mom had gathered me and Keith under her arms, lain flat, and then lain on top of us with arms outstretched to bravely over us.

One of the highlights of the war was when the Canadian soldiers occupied the buildings of a private girls school in the little town. The students and staff were evacuated inland. Keith and I and our friends played happily in the school fields and chatted with the soldiers. One told us he was an "Indian" and his name was Archie. We were very impressed at having spoken to a real "Indian."

When the grass was finally cut, The kids would push hay into the shape of Spitfires, or tanks, and invent great war manoeuvres. The soldiers were pretty amused; one told Keith and our dad, "The girl is a real sergeant major."

I also told how our little gang had done scrump (stealing) raids for apples and pears from the unattended private school orchard. Sometimes we would flee away, laughing and shouting. One time we leaped over a low stone wall, only to find the drop was considerably deeper on the other side.

Once, British soldiers also played a part in our young lives. One day we came trudging through the town on a long march, stopping for a rest on the grass at the end of the street. Keith and I ran home to get water and lemonade for them. The soldiers probably would have preferred something else, but our mother offered big jugs of lemonade.

Still another encounter with soldiers was very different. While my little gang was prying around an area where we shouldn't have been, a soldier asked us if we had seen a bunch of soldiers nearby. We hadn't but decided to go looking for us. As we peeped over a small embankment, we were horrified to see a whole army racing toward us over a nearby field. The little gang turned and fled in terror, though we knew the soldiers were "our guys."

*

I spoke of another weird episode that occurred when the family were living in a tiny village in the midlands. My mother was a cook at private school that had been evacuated from the coast while our dad was in Coventry as an air raid warden.

Without Keith or I hearing it, a German plane crashed at night by a little stream near the school. It was believed the pilot fell into the water and drowned. By the time we got up in the morning, the place was swarming with soldiers who'd set up a guard over what was left of the plane. I could not remember whether they stayed in huts on the grounds or had tents. But they set up a huge wooden frame on which they wove camouflage nets; we even let her weave in a few bits of green and khaki stuff.

The soldiers spent a lot of time carving things from the plane's plastic windows. One made an ornament to give to the school's headmistress when we left.

Sometimes, during the early years of the war, the kids

were issued identification tags. They were made of a compressed cardboard and imprinted with our identity number. We quickly learned them. I remembered hers: EJNI 2904. Keith, who was born twenty minutes after me was one rung down the ladder: EJNI2905. We were very proud of our I.D. discs that we were supposed to wear all the time. But then we found out why we had to do that. A school friend told us: "It's for knowing who you are if you get dug out dead from a bombed house." Somehow the discs lost our charm after that.

Our family followed our dad to Coventry when he was transferred with Civil Defence. It was after the big bombing which destroyed lots of the city. The family was housed in a flat which had suffered bomb damage. I recalled leaning on the fireplace mantel only to have it give way, cutting my hand.

Although we had few air raids, we were scared out of our wits one night shortly after the siren had sounded. The air was filled with a sound like immense gunfire and swoosh, unlike the normal anti-aircraft. Our dad had his helmet on outside. The rest of the family ran to crouch in the hallway, again with our brave mother standing over her children with her arms spread out. Finally the noise stopped and Dad came back in with a big grin—a new type of rocket gun had been installed along with the ack-ack guns. The racket was from the rockets that burst into box-like formation around enemy planes. So we could all breathe again.

Another time, closer to the end of the war, the family was back visiting in Seaford. We twins' cousin, Derek, a few years older than us, asked if we had seen the new German V1 and V2 buzz bombs. We hadn't.

Again a siren went. The twins hung out the bedroom window.

"Here comes one," Derek shouted.

We heard what sounded like an airborne motor bike. We watched, rooted in excited fear. A long cigar-shaped object with small fins at the back came into view. There was a red light glowing at the back. Suddenly the light went out. "What do we do now?" we asked Derek.

He was going along the hall leading to the stairs. "Run like hell," he shouted, and we did—to the backyard shelter. The bomb exploded more or less harmlessly, in mid-air. The bombs did real damage when we landed and exploded.

One of the biggest banes of "Keith and my War" was the air raid shelter. At first the family had only Anderson shelters, usually in the backyard, a very miserable place to be in an Anderson shelter, sunk into the ground, and completely covered with piles of dirt. We were cold and usually damp. We did not feel the least bit secure.

Sometimes we would run into the cupboard under the staircase. At least we didn't have to run outside again, and it was warm.

The shelter we dreaded the most was the Morrison

shelter. It was in the family sitting room, a huge thing like a big steel table, which had mattresses on the floor, and also on top, so we could sleep if the air raid went on long. It was constructed in such a way that, once everyone was inside, we were more or less lying down. A long grid was pulled across the opening, presumably to keep out debris should the house collapse.

We, a family of five grew to seven when our eldest sister married a young Canadian airman who became a prisoner of the war, and I came home with our baby. Everyone together in the shelter was a thing of claustrophobic horror.

One night, the siren went. One aunt and uncle, plus a young cousin, where visiting. Into the shelter we all went, laid out like cord wood. The twins' dad and uncle stayed outside, thrusting our heads under when the guns were going off. All were thankful there were too many of us for the grid to be put into place and close us in.

Keith and I often went to school the next day wearing the clothes we'd slept in. We felt and looked like a crumpled-looking lot, but then so did everyone else attending school.

We were with our father and mother in Brighton, where we were then living. We (the twins) were thirteen. Then the war ended in July, we turned fourteen, left school, and went to work. We had grown up. We were little kids in 1939. In May 1945, we were adults.

When I think back to Keith and Lesley's loss of childhood

caused by the war, I wonder if that, plus other traumatic times in their lives, contributed to their dementia. I think about how Lesley gave her all to make life in Norway House residential school more humane and meaningful for the girls in residence, only to be included in the never-ending punishing blame, alongside me, first as a naïve, nineteen-year-old boys' supervisor, later a teacher.

Tantamount to our decision to adopt, Lesley suffered a miscarriage while we lived in Norway House. After the procedure at the local hospital, a nurse or doctor abruptly said to Lesley, "You know you lost your baby. It was a boy." What followed was that she could no longer give birth.

Lesley and I adopted two boys of Cree ancestry and a girl of Kutchin ancestry.

Years later, the wear and tear on Lesley and me—most certainly for being blamed for our part in the "Sixties Scoop,"(placement of native children in non-native homes). Despite our care and devotion to our adopted loved ones—we were left hopelessly distraught.

Could this blame be a contributor to Lesley's pro-longed depression, leading to mental and physical pain she suffered eventually swallowed up by the black hole "dementia"? Cumulatively, could the many moves, demanding constant readjusting and adapting added to the stress? (See the list of places where we, as a family lived.) Could Lesley and Keith's beginnings as children of war also contribute to their Dementia?

Chapter 5: The Power of Spirit Lake Park

I felt the loss of a very intelligent, empathetic, competent woman whom I loved. Her death left me with the question: Should I go on living? Lesley's life had given meaning and purpose to mine. We had shared so much, including experiencing the power of Spirit Island Park. So I felt compelled to begin my journey by revisiting the power of that Park.

The park has the power to get a person thinking about what really matters. If one persists in circling the park's lake, not out of habit or obsession, but as a way of connecting to the power of nature, one may find the experience most revealing over time. Each experience gained through the senses stimulates not only the imagination, but much more. Trips around the park bring about journeys into the mind, picking out thoughts, memories, ideas, and dreams. The power of nature does that if we are open to it.

For the park's power evokes inspiring truths in stories that reconnect one with nature and people inspiring to live on.

Chosen Goslings
(a metaphor related to the children
Lesley and I adopted)

The water splashed and the winged air movers, including geese, asserted their place in nature's scheme of things and so it holds true, when one tugs at a thing in nature, he finds it is attached to the rest of the world. Those attached in the park, the water birds, like geese, ducks and gulls, are busy through the day, unlike soaring hawks and eagles that rarely spread their wings early in the morning. They usually wait until the sun warms the air enough to catch the rising currents.

What a picture! Staring up into the sky, one can marvel at the gliding grace and nodding necks of the predators whose natural mission to kill can overcome mesmerizing prey using aerial displays. Oh, if only humans could demonstrate such finesse. But whether we like it or not, in nature, the emphasis is in what is, rather than what ought to be.

That's true for park visitors who need resign

themselves to the raucous squawking on Spirit Island Lake, the ridiculous peeping from adolescent geese, who should by now offer decent honks, and geese droppings; We also must share space with sociable geese lounging on the golf course, and the intimidating hesitation of geese arrogantly strutting about the paths.

Geese, wearing down-filled vests, do make their presence known with nasal voices, V-ing to or hustling fro after gorging farmers' grain. The kerfuffle of noisy efforts intensifies when grey, heavy skies, ice-crystallized air, and open frigid water succumbs to glassy ice crusts. Then anxious geese raise bellies and slap the water to keep it open, while honking complaints. So it is that when the lake gets congested with geese there doesn't seem to be any room left on the water for others circling, trying to land. The noises of others, who have already laid claim to water rights, deafens.

One person taking in the drama asked another, "What's going on?"

The others "Those on the water are telling the ones in the air to SCRAM."

Sadness about seeing the necessity of this annual repeat performances just doesn't enter the minds of most park visitors, for just as nature packs away one suit of colourful clothing she brings out another, repeating it four times in its park living room, So the geese, along with other migrating birds, sometimes grounded by low ceilings, other times free to fly high through open skies, yearly remind us of our need to adjust to changing conditions. That's life!

But sometimes these athletic, gung-ho geese take the easy way out and succumb to becoming feathered couch potatoes. no longer park in long lines, like beads in for migration mood, but rather throw their lot in with other pesky birds.

"Sometimes birds learn to exploit modern ecological alternatives.

Gulls thrive on garbage dumps and migrant shore birds frequent sewage beds (Wild Goose Chase Inc. Blog. October 26, 2020)

"DO NOT FEED THE GEESE" is the point.

Migrant birds like geese can become dependent on handouts from people and thus stop foraging. Waiting for food to come to them leaves them too weak to migrate, even if wanted that. Mouldy bread and fruit, instead of natural foods, leftovers from from home "feed the geese" amuse both geese and people. This is bad news for geese. It causes them to hang around instead of migrating as they're supposed to do.

It seems these waterfowl know they are safe from hunters when plunking down on the park's Spirit Lakefront. That primitive instinctive behaviour is not only something to behold, even though it's a predictable annual event, but it leaves human spectators with the unfinished business of trying to answer the questions of children less familiar with the performances. When the birds on the water arena are in a restless mood and it looks like there ready to head south how do they know when that moment has come? Who decides? one leader or more than one?

Why the "V" formation? Why don't they just take off, each doing its own thing? A student in a Sociology 101 course gave an answer: Watching geese in formation, the birds taking turns in the lead position, is an example of what should happen in human groups. There is a need to spell off leaders, giving them breaks by taking backseat positions, at least for a while.

"One other, an ornithology student, familiar "*Feathered Life*" by Garry .Kaiser answered in another way.

A few birds, like geese and pelicans so frequently seen flying in 'V' formation or in straight lines have the advantage of flying that way because each bird behind the one in front of him/her gets a little bit of lift from the flap of the bird it follows, who creating a vacuum, makes the upstroke easier for the next. All the academic mental gymnastics still leaves most who frequent the park with a haunting feeling that there is more that touch us on a deeper level when in company with nature's flying miracles.

Two geese unlike the others in the flock preened and proudly displayed their recently hatched, confused-looking goslings.

In the following weeks, more and more ganders left females to raise their broods as single mothers. The ganders seemed to assume they had done their bit. But some mothers just couldn't cope with big families. Some young goslings, smaller and weaker than most, just couldn't figure out how to feed and stay out of trouble. Sooner or later they die snatched up by grasping claws of diving predators or yanked underwater by sharp-toothed fish. Even if grow rapidly in days ahead, they'd be less likely to keep up with the flock, having had a poor start in life. If by chance they did, would they, so ill-prepared, survive hunters blue steel blasts to circle and glide to peaceful ends?

Those questions mingled with the moist mist of dawn while under-threatened mothers and diminished broods try to shorten the honking distance between other mothers' flocks frantically trying to save their gaggle of curious peepers.

Deep voices and gently swaying necks, with strength in numbers, the moms seemed reassured eventually that no more harm could come to them or their broods.

Among the single moms was a childless goose begging to raise a gosling. Her eggs hadn't hatched that year, She longed to see peeping balls of feathers grow into splashing, awkward, voice-changing adolescents, and finally into strong, business-like hissing, honking Canadian geese.

As mother with proud gander, she would take on

responsibility to love, provide for, and protect her brood.

So much happened after that. The gander had run a flight school for beginners who hadn't yet earned their wings and had no idea how to fly the "V" formation. It was that year his lifelong partner hatched no eggs. Having no hope for another hatching that year or ever, the couple tried to adopt.

A question asked by an onlooker was this: did the would-be parents swimming among the big bunch of newly hatched have preferences?

It looked like it didn't matter what size, colour, or amount of fatherless goslings were showed as they bobbed about. Any three would do and receive unconditional love and attention.

There was yet one thing left to do though. The adopting couple had to pass some tests to prove worthy of bringing the adopted up to flying speed to have what it took to fly south with the flock. Feeding was important. Could would-be parents get the attention of the goslings they had in mind to adopt, to learn how to find just the right weedy spots, dip bills into the water to feed? Would the gander stay around to help the mother with goslings? Did the new soon-to-be parents have a call that the goslings would pay attention to, even when the little rascals mere too busy doing their own things distant from Mom and dad? Would the parents demonstrate honks and other parent sounds that could be sorted out as different from the rest of the flock members? All the questions had to be answered before the adopted parents could takes charge of their new brood.

So, before the couple could swim away with three goslings, the mothers in charge of the flocks day care had to still wave beaks in approval. In the meantime, the parents-to-be had permission to swim about nearby.

Weeks passed. But then the day care bosses waved necks, an invitation for the couple to swim close for goose talk. It appeared that the day care bosses that had waved had three other goslings in mind than the three wanted. The couple were led to three others. The day care bosses waved necks, splashed the water with their wings, circled about in the water, wings dipping, all to entice the couple to accept three others instead of the ones they'd chosen.

The couple passed all the tests, but the day care bosses had chosen for them. These were bigger, older, and better behaviour-wise. Was that it?

The onlooker to the drama wondered whether the new parents were viewed as too old; maybe it was thought they'd not be able to survive the hunters' gun blasts through the years it would take to raise goslings. No, it wasn't that. For the flock would somehow care for the little ones left orphaned if worst came to worst. Besides, the time to fly south and leave the park haven was months away.

The couple, not wanting to give the impression they

were too old to care for little ones, put their hearts and souls into demonstrating excellent swimming, flying, feeding, and fending-off-intruder skills. They swooped, dipped, and dived, performing extraordinary aerial acrobatics and hissing loudly, making a downright nuisance of themselves, pecking and poking neighbours. They did, indeed, look sincere in their intentions,

Finally, those making the big decision threw up wings in surrender, stopped dragging web feet through the water, and nodded with their bills to where the couple were to pick up their chosen goslings.

The couple wagged tails, waved long necks, touched blue bills, chattered, gave polite, sedate honks, ran across the water, gracefully lifting off with the morning sun shining on their white jaw patches, broad-fanned black-and-grey wings effortlessly flapping, signalling satisfaction and pleasure.

Soon the two hovered over the mud-banked creek. Its murky water, like glass, mirrored a dark reflection of the two dropping onto the glassy surface perhaps an omen of dark days ahead .Three little fuzz balls paddled under the bridge, gently herded by a matronly goose.

At last, the moment arrived; the couple would unite with their brood..

The onlooker thought, *Well that's it, they shall live happily ever after.* But then the matronly escort had the last word before disappearing under the bridge and out of sight. One of the babies looked sickly. The onlooker imagined, in watching the escort splashing and wing gestures, that the escort could be warning the little one suffered a chronic bird chest condition. Causing goose parents, to have their wings full trying to keep that sickly one alive. One could hear a little dry cough and see the little fellow labouring to catch his breath. But despite the warning, the couple, without question wanted the little gosling to love. He had such a sad look while pointing his little peak in the direction of the couple. His tiny web feet paddled frantically while he struggled to reach the circle of safety around the couple.

The other two goslings were already nestled close to their new mom and dad. The sickly gosling perked up as the two grownups embraced him, but when seeking to join he family in the big water under the bridge, the little urchin began peeping pathetically, leaving the new parents to return once again to embrace him reassuringly.

The couple with goslings set out to re-join their own flock far down the lake.

It wasn't an easy journey. The little one's web feet sometimes got tangled while hugging the shoreline, ready at any time to huddle in the shadows of the rocks lining the lake. Where the parent geese could break the surface of the water at a pre-flight gate, their little charges had to struggle along, looking very vulnerable.

Through sunrise and sunset and into the cool darkness of

night, the family warily made its way. When the sun lifted its head out of the grey morning haze to cast a warm glow on the birds' backs, they finally arrived to be greeted warmly as the sun.

The mom and dad, now so elated, having their own brood safely home, lifted their bodies into the air, soaring, dipping wings, circling, honking a delightful duet. Then having roused the drowsy, sleeping heads from under wings, swooped over their own and landed, coasting up to their goslings like float planes.

When humans would wave and cast gesturing reflections on glassy surfaces surroundings the dock, the tired little goslings and parents were greeted by a nose-blowing flock splashing, tail-waggling gaggle of geese. So bent on well-wishing, these well-wishers, embarrassed almost lost their graceful water-sifting dignity, finding the five family members feather touching, diplomatic honking, peeps, and web feet wiggling that worked well in gaining acceptance by the flock. But one energetic gosling, the older of the three, just couldn't put his best foot forward. He pleasantly surprised his mom and dad goose by trying to fly with a few feathered baby wing stumps. The youngster, when not stirring up the waters to imitate his adopted parents, stirred things up by pestering the patient ganders who now and then hissed and pecked at him. Eventually not getting anywhere with the grownups, he spun his fluffy body about, and, twisting and turning, elbowed his sister and brother, peeping and pestering, forcing them to scurry over to their mothers.

The honking orchestra, familiar to human bystanders, settled in to give renditions of its usual domestic bliss. Then feathers would fly. Why? Because the little guy who, having swum with wing limbs tucked under his feathers, looking lonely and bored, nudged his way into the crowd. Then, when given a gentle push or two, lost his temper, hissing attacked the biggest gander who had his back turned. The little gosling just couldn't let things be. He just had to keep pushing to see how far he could go, to see what would happen if he disturbed the way things were in the flock. He even nipped the tail feathers of another mighty big gander that usually stood guard when the others had our heads down nibbling grass, sleeping, or gossiping. The mischievous gosling's mother often swam over to him to let him snuggle up to her, but he'd push her away, showing no affection and distancing himself from her.

It wasn't long before the gosling's mom and dad began fussing about, honking, chasing, and herding back that restless one while trying to soothe the ruffled feathers of those he troubled.

He was a cute little thing, and the onlooker often saw some female auntie-like birds fuss over him. But the water was brown and tepid and things were heating up in the usually sociable flock, with the trouble generated by the new family's unhappy gosling. It looked like things just wouldn't work out where the troubled family swam.. Then the onlooker, concerned for the newly formed family, was relieved. He saw a big gander lead the family away from the flock. He led the family of five in his wake, down the lake to where another flock noisily neighboured together.

By then the family looked very weary. The onlooker imaged the family members might feel more comfortable with the new flock. It looked like a real mix of birds of all shapes, sizes, and shades of grey mixed with white. There were also many ducks, a real mix swimming among the geese. The newly adopted parents were of one breed of geese with adopted goslings. So perhaps in the new flock things would work out better. Maybe. Though it looked like the troubled little gosling suddenly realized the other two, his new sister and brother, weren't going anywhere, despite his peeping, hissing, and other throaty sounds that together sounded like "Goslings, go home."

He put his slow head down, sorrowfully swimming about, giving the onlooker the idea that the little creature realized he'd have to share with his new brother and sister for the attention of their parents.

That first night among the second flock, all but one of five melded themselves into sleeping shapes, looking like pebbles or rocks. Throughout the night and into the early morning hours, the troubled one's brother slept almost under the wings of his mother. But that didn't last long. Soon he feather-puffed his way onto the slimy weeded space between some shore rocks. His mother retrieved him, nudging him back to the safety of the flock. This drifting away and escorting back went on for hours, despite his mother's efforts to limit his restless movements away from the circle of safety.

The little urchin gosling, unlike his brother and sister gosling, looked bedraggled. His feather coat looked mottled. His little head looked flea-bitten, and his gangling legs and web feet toed inward, a sight for sore eyes. Veteran ganders of many flights through shotgun pellet-sprayed corridors and hail thrashings couldn't look worse than the troubled gosling. Still the onlooker said to himself, "What a beautiful creature!"

The ragged little gosling continued his restless sleeping habits in his new home. Many suns rose and set, and in time he began hoisting himself onto the water-lapped slippery rocks on the shore. He and his brother used nature's playground equipment, rocks and reeds, weeds, and the odd floating log to test their strength. The troubled one, though a bit smaller, used his speed and cunning in play. But in the eyes of bystanders, he often didn't play fair. Maybe by goose rules that was okay. But the younger, whose voice was changing from a meek peep to a raspy broken honk, let it be known, having got most of the cuffs and bumps from his brother, that he was frustrated.

Yet, the two did show mutual interests enjoying the interesting mix of noise bill vibrations that ricocheted off the rocks, trees, which they tried to imitate. Though tail wagging, stirring up the water, also delighted, they enjoyed making noisy nose sounds punctuated by burping.

Other adolescent geese shared the water with the mallard ducks who often came and played with them. The onlooker thought the visitor to the adopted parents' patch of water seemed surprised, as did the grown-ups when the older of the three youngsters did something unusual for a goose. Seeing a dog on the path by the water's edge, instead of saying *"Woof, woof"* which in itself would be unusual for a goose, he stretched open his beak, and out came what sounded like *"Kingmiuk."* The surprised onlooker remembered that word was an approximation of the Inuit word for dog. He thought, well, that little creature is honking in Canadian, as the name of his species indicates. Though perhaps that would be more appropriate coming out of the throat of a snow goose, rather than a Canadian Goose. Suppose the little creature had been by a Snow Goose passing through? Would he have spent more time in the Arctic, assimilated into the local Snow Goose culture? Maybe he'd inter-marry and raise Canadian Snow Geese. That wouldn't be too far-fetched. But, then again, would he be accepted by his adopted parents' geese family? One wonders.

The onlooker saw the mother of the adopted three showing concern and fear for the safety of her brood, especially one dark moonlight night when the stillness was broken by the sound of powerful predator's wings above the water. The mother began frantically swimming and honking, searching for her three. Her two teenaged males wandered off on their own more frequently, foraging further away each day. Now, though, wasn't the time to assert independence. They no doubt might have gone to their deaths under the claws of night prowlers lurking overhead, as many had before, had it not been for a mother, who spotted one, then the other two, and nudged each back into the shelter of the rocks.

The mother goose looked agitated, not only when conscious of dangers without, but also those within her three goslings. The one troubled bedraggled little one was falling behind the family during outings in search of food among the weeds and other water plants. The gosling would shake his head as if to rid himself of something that didn't belong within him. He would repeatedly give a half-hearted honk, but it was as if he didn't give a hoot. His heart just wasn't in it. He was obviously ill, becoming weaker. Others with the same symptoms often died, and their putrefying bodies floated about like dead fish belly-up on the froth along the lake shore.

The mother goose, somehow seemed to know she couldn't cure her sick one. Leading her three along the shore, stopping often to let her sick one catch up, she finally swam into the shallows with her brood. Humans passing by along the water's edge may have noticed the mother with two healthy goslings, and a sickly one nudged by her onto the lake's boat ramp. The mother didn't look surprised or concerned when a passing human on the path gently picked up the sickly gosling, cradled it in her hands, warmed it inside her jacket and headed for her car. The mother goose didn't seem surprised either when, weeks later, the same human returned and gently set her absentee gosling, now well, back in the water to join the other two feeding. Nor was the mother surprised when her now well gosling wagged its tail flapped its wings, twisted its neck and head in swaying motions, shyly giving each of its siblings, a gentle peck on their necks.

The onlooker thought, *Well, I'll be darned. Have other feathered friends connected in similar, profound mysterious ways with humans?*

The raw instinct to survive played out every moment on the lake and by the shore. Dogs took humans for walks along the path bordering the shore. Geese and ducks loitered and casually pecked and dipped under for morsels of bugs and choice bits of weed. Some geese flew or scrambled and hopped over the rocks to strut about, arching long necks down to stretch and nibble at the grass under the watchful eye of a towering-necked gander.

A dog dancing merrily down the path might come to

a lurching halt, lean forward, sometimes bark, sniff the air and twang its leash to get at the geese. The geese, not wanting to appear undignified, head up, slowly land-paddled toward the water, refusing to lose graceful composure. Where dogs often acted uncouth, the geese portrayed a royal presence till each hit the water, and with a frenzy flurry of flapping wings, distanced themselves from dogs and human companions.

While the open water gave the gun-shy geese an opportunity to feel safe, the boulders lining the lake gave dogs and humans a chance to play the game of hop and slip, lose balance, and even sprain or break an ankle or leg. Attentive to keeping a footing they often lost all interest in departing ducks or geese.

Dogs can be a blessing or a curse, the onlooker thought. He remembered being in the north where dogs sometimes ran wild, sources of danger to children. Many local dogs ran in packs, and when the winds blew strong sometimes became vicious. Stories were told of packs killing, or maiming children.

Dogs frequenting the park were usually well controlled, less a danger to people than to geese. Once before, when the father gander had gone off with the other ganders, leaving the mother and goslings to fend for themselves, a huge, long-haired husky sniffed around the water's edge. Though it did not venture onto the boulders, it did do what huskies do. It howled and howled, getting the attention of the gander, who hadn't heard that sound up close before. His only acquaintance was with hunting dogs, especially retrievers, some who couldn't tell the difference between a dead or alive duck or goose. The gander eventually lost interest in the big dog, and the dog lost interest in the gander and his family. But it didn't lose interest in what sled dogs do. It yanked and pulled on its leash, imagining it pulled a sled. Its petite female owner all but flew through the air as he took her for a run down the path

After the gander left, its mate found a safe secluded spot by the water running under the path. There, like any mom with dad away, kept her thee close by, watching play often ending up in feathers flying, and murky water muddying up feathered coats.

The onlooker thought about the parents, where one was often away, like the gander that'd left the goose to care for the goslings. He imagined that if geese could think like human creatures, they might have recalled, as he did, that much happened when one parent was away from the family.

He thought back to one family he knew about. The geese, the park, and the lake reminded him of it and what each member had faced. The park and its inhabitants continued to evoke other thoughts of other times and places.

Stories as Metaphors to Visit While Grieving

Lesley and I wrote these stories together long before her death. In my grief work leading up to me determined to live on after her death, I found it necessary to revisit these story metaphors to get back on board encouraged to complete oneness with others celebrating life to the fullest.

Perhaps others, like me, who grieve will find light in despair, and inspiration to live on beyond a loved one's death from dementia

The Unwelcomed Visitor

The lamp light shone onto the side of the rough-barked aging tree. Beyond, down the path narrowed by the golf course and Japanese garden chain link fences, walked a lone figure. A sudden flapping noise above his head, somewhere in the twisted branches of a tree, stopped him cold. He listened and looked. Then, hearing only the spewing of water into the frigid air above the golf course pond, he shrugged and began his shuffle toward the opening onto the parking lot bordered by a busy road.

The next day, the walker passed a couple coming up on the mouth of the path. It was six a.m. The breeze rippled the water. Ducks that had hobbled about the day before hid in the shadowed scum near the rocks.

The couple paused and pointed. At what? The walker

looked. What was that on the tree top? It looked big for a flicker or crow, and it wasn't an owl. It couldn't be!

"Yes, an eagle," said the couple.

"That's strange," said the walker. "Must have lost its way."

"No, I heard some at the other park's lake. That's nowhere near as big as this one. The city is having some eagle visitors."

A week's worth of sun rising and setting saw the walker frequently stopping and asking couples if they'd seen the eagle in flight. That yellow-billed frowning tufted head dignified its body, balanced motionlessly high above the walker's head. Did anyone photograph that intruder in the act of swooping off with a gosling in its cruel talons?

The walker hadn't heard. All he knew, one day stopping by the tree where the eagle had perched he saw eagle had gone.

He thought back to his childhood, remembering walking a wider path, a road, seeing the Case company tractor globe symbol topped off with an eagle, wings folded. As an imaginative child, he'd hoped that it too would spread its mighty wings and take flight. It never did. The disappointments of life accumulated in his memory clusters, to await the coming of an eagle or nature's other surprises. Thus, the present never escaped the past.

Lone Wild Goose

A lone wild goose seemed frozen in nature's photo frame. Water lapped at its tuxedo-dressed chest. But unlike a debonair, proud in command presence, its plaintive, pathetic vibrations moved through the still air, reaching across the water to Spirit Lake Park and to throngs of gossiping noisy couples.

A walker on the lake path stopped. There was a disturbance above his head. He searched the heavy blanket of clouds; a low-flying flock broke through into sight, descended, and landed across the lake, among the early birds' gossiping flock.

The walker looked at a bird without its mate swimming apart from the flock. He thought about how, like the lonely bird, a person who, having lost his/her spouse through death, no longer enjoys the company of friends who knew them as a couple. Now it was different. In the company of couples, the goose, too, was the odd one out. Friends didn't quite know what to do with this survivor, and the bereaved one's new awkwardness showed, for the bird's mate's death affected his place in the flock, if there was one.

Getting Old

Someone once said, "To be any earthly good when one gets old, one needs to forget to remember." How so? Keeping one's head screwed on right means paying attention to the here and now. True useful wisdom for the young comes from sharing years lived: "The more sand that has escaped from the hourglass of our life, the clearer one should see through it." True also that "Old wood best to burn, old wine to drink, old friends to trust, and old authors to be read." True again: It's been asked in history by Francis Bacon and years later by Rose Kennedy "Birds sing after a storm. Why shouldn't people feel as free to delight in whatever sunlight remains for them." anon

But, as demonstrated by many vigorous old-in-years, but not in body and mind, fast hoofing it down he park paths, laughing and playing with children, no one need wallow in the tepid waters of philosophy. For, the active in the park surely must believe, "If you carry your childhood with you, your willpower never becomes older." "Age is an issue of mind over matter. If you don't mind it, it doesn't matter."

Though many aged don't sing that out loud as convincing lyrics, many who are park regulars say, "Keep putting one foot in front of the other," head down, doggedly determined. Perhaps we remember what Charles M. Schulz, author of Peanuts cartoons once said, thinking there is no time to waste, life is precious. "Just remember, once you're over the hill, you begin to pick up speed."

Some others may have had the same thought. So, as couples gathered together, not "remembering back then," but despite canes, wheelchairs, or scooters risked frequenting the park, looking very attentive, focused, keenly interested, not in personal well-being so much as what was still out there to challenge. They somehow latched onto the idea that, as Henry Wadsworth Longfellow said, "To be seventy years old is like climbing the Alps. You reach a snow-crowned summit and see behind you the deep valley stretching miles and miles away, and before you other summits higher and whiter, which you may have strength to climb, or may not. Then you sit down and meditate and wonder which it will be."

So the bystander, viewing the human activity and being long-in-the-tooth himself, comes to the conclusion that a person is still young as long as he/she are seeking something.

Sadly, viewing human activity in the park, he often sees evidence of that idea not being heard even by those young in years.

Abandoned

Oh, that hurts. Gee, I don't want to get up, but I got to uncurl those toes. What if I just relax, and start by bending my knees, then work my way down. Doesn't help. The warm blankets better than cold when my feet hit the floor. What time is it? Darn. The clock slipped off the side table. Never went off. Right, I didn't set it. Amazing, I can see with the night light, it's five. Oh, still can't uncurl my toes. Got to sit up, stand up, push down. Forget the slippers. Bathroom first. It feels some better. Oh, it's indeed better now. Go back to bed. No, can't take a chance, better stay up. Gee, now I got a bloody kink in my back. Can't be kidney stones. Feels like muscle spasms, maybe. Hate to turn the bathroom light on, always have to squeeze my eyes tight, then open us slowly. Better, I guess, than a kink in my foot or toes. The message in the mirror doesn't help my disposition. The Health Watch on TV says sagging stomachs are not good for the heart. What time is it now? It's not light yet. The exercise bike, that's a possibility. No, I said I'd start running around the park lake. Maybe across the two bridges and around the lagoon, better dress in my sweats, yes. This is different, haven't felt so determined about restoring my body. I could try to get into those things in the closet, should have given to the Sally Ann. But still could try to get into them, easier when I was in better shape.

Well, it soon will be light. Don't want to wake anyone though. Want to surprise them with the kettle on, toast smells when I get back. We'll be pleased I got out and did that walk. Where are those runners, the new ones, A clerk showed me how to slip the laces through the loops at the top. I'll be just like those athletes running the lake paths and able to talk at the same time, unlike those clumping along, gasping for air. But like them I'll get over that. Now the new runners. Sit on a chair to put them on. Big decision this early in the morning. Undo the laces a little more. A shoehorn doesn't seem the thing for these.

Well, should I leave the light on above the stove? The only thing is, it reminds me to get someone to fix the stove fan. A bunch things to do. I wish I hadn't signed off on this new house. I like the smell of new, but it's the little things, just as bad as kink in the toes.

It's light enough now. I won't drive to the park. A couple of blocks to warm up. That will stretch the stiffness out. When I get by that long stretch of chain fence keeping people off the golf course, I'll pick up speed. It seems to cool down a bit, and the grass is wet. Better stay on the sidewalk and path. This is good. Better tummy breathe from the bottom of the lungs. Better than top. Something about the warm-up bit, can get to feel empty, not just stomach, but the whole business. It's cleansing. Well, which way should I go, the long way running by the golf course or past the guns to my left, and swing around by the picnic table water and washrooms? That's the way, and finish off with the long bit.

This is weird, I thought I'd meet someone by now. I look like a runner, dressed just so, I'll just walk. Must be the first one here. Well, there's the floating docks, bench, pier. I'll keep going. No one in the parking lot. Not one truck. I must have beaten all here. What's that over there by the boat ramp, the space between the rocks, on the grass there. It's piles, two of them,. A couple of ducks? There are usually more around here. Clothes, what the? Shoes, a pair, flannel shirt, faded jeans, torn, greasy-like. Who'd leave those, all neatly piled. No undershorts though. Why did I think that? But the other lot, not tidily piled, scattered pullover shirt, pants out of style, no shoes, jacket near the path, all thrown about as if stripped off a body in a rush. A couple of bottles, not "this is Canadian." Bigger, maybe whisky. Near the rocks. But this stuff must belong to two guys. No one in sight.

Oh my God! Gee, I wish I had my cell phone. Got to get to one. Run! Got to get back to the lake side. No, run! Wake up someone in the house across from the parking lot. Phone 9-1-1. I think the two drowned. Don't know who. But for sure that must have happened. But if I phone, will others come along, see the clothes, and make the same call? Should I leave a note with the clothes? Ridiculous, get going, get going!

*

Some Big Questions

Shortly after finding the abandoned clothing, evidence of a tragedy, he sat on a park bench. His precious thoughts about nature's sensuality faded, replaced by the big questions of life, which are: Who am I? Why am I here? Where am I going? He had often heard that the death of a loved one or friend kicks us into gear to ask those questions. Now he was caught up in that tough struggle for answers. He began by remembering that he was in the park, the home of other creatures like himself. That prompted another question: What makes humans human and birds and animals different?

People big and small passed by his park bench. He thought, *Curious creatures we are, herd animals. Once we had hair all over our bodies, that's why we get goose bumps. So we are something like all animals, same beginnings.* Some highfalutin scientist he saw on TV's *Nature of Things* talked about culture being transmitted through the genes, with one difference being between animals and humans. We humans have the power to direct evolution, whereas birds and others have to just go along with the changes. He also talked about the question of nature or nurture—which is it? Do some people's kids do the damnedest things because we were born bad, screwed-up genes maybe, or did the grownups that looked after them screw up in the raising? Or did the kids they hung around with have the greatest say about whether they would be bad or good? One big difference between birds and animals and humans is that the other creatures, unlike humans, don't think about these things, they just do what comes naturally, and there just isn't good or bad for them, there just is.

The thing about we humans is we "see the world not as it is, but as we are." Something else about humans: We each have our own minds, and so not everyone sees things the same way, nor do we learn the same way—unlike animals and birds. You take two or more people who size up a situation, or see an accident, each sees it differently.

Pondering over that idea, he asks: Suppose a flock of geese flew over some humans in the park that were fussing over something that happened. Would each gander see things differently? And so on through the flock, each goose or gander sizing up what's even and conclude differently? Would we, like geese on landing, debate who was right and who was wrong? He didn't suppose so. Maybe that's one advantage humans have over other creatures. How does it go? "One point of view gives a one-dimensional world." Humans have many points of view, and we sure let others know about them.

The park bench sitter thought some more about this and decided humans have a whole lot of other tendencies, some that even get us into a whole lot of trouble, or worse, tie us in knots inside. Take young people, for instance; from an older person's point of view, they get so hung up. As psychologists say, in preoccupations: loneliness, resentment, anger, disillusionment, self-doubt, aimlessness, and so on.

Maybe young people could learn from an experiment where a big, hungry fish is put into a fish tank, a glass partition halving the tank. On one side swims a juicy little minnow. The huge fish charges toward the little fish to gobble it, only to bump its nose against the glass partition. It backs up, takes another run at it, and again bumps his nose on the partition. Over and over it does this, but each time puts a little less effort into it, thinking, *what the heck, it's impossible.* The big fish finally gives up. Then the glass separation is removed, and sadly the big fish starves to death.

That whole idea about how people can get discouraged, rebuffed, and give up seems to be something that we humans have in common with other creatures. People, unlike birds and animals, do have the power to get out of that trap. One can have the power to go on shyly scratching our way through life, or step out, risk, or mentally retreat back into the womb where it's warm, cozy, and safe and "do nothing for nobody." We could decide whether we want to be pushed or pulled along through life, jump through hoops for others, have little control of our own lives, or end up like puppets with others pulling the strings, jerking us around. Then when, hurting inside, fed up with it all, go around grinning on the outside, crying on the inside.

The park bench sitter thought about a whole lot of other stuff that had to do with how he and others were wired—that is, what makes humans tick. He thought about the business of mating. How that's both a human and animal need. He thought about competitiveness—how that's a built-in human trait. But he didn't think animals and birds were so caught up in that, except a need for food, or when the opposite sex was around.

Just then, a friend he often had coffee with came along, stopped, sat down, and away the two went chewing the rag about people. Why we do what we do, and what we should do, and don't do. They tossed questions and answers about as if playing catch with a ball.

"Why is it when I start to pass someone, they speed up all of a sudden? It is as if that person thought I wanted to challenge him to a drag race. That's damn silly, that when I glance over to eye the person I'm trying to pass, he turns out to look like my granddad, who's dead!"

"And what about the tailgaters? We give them time and space to pass, and they still stay up our backsides. I haven't seen those geese flying in formations acting that way. They seem to have more sense than that."

"Something else I noticed about some people, in fact, I think it may be even one of my hang-ups: When I was a kid, I had this thing about not stepping on a crack in the sidewalk, and, like some others that I know, I always have to go back and forth trying a door repeatedly to make sure it's locked. Once doesn't seem enough to reassure me it is. Crazy thing, I'm out the door in the car and I feel I've got to make sure. Even now, here I am sitting with you in the park and I'm thinking, did I turn off the stove, the lights, and flush the toilet?"

"That is a dilemma. Maybe you should think about what one guy said: 'Life can be understood only backwards, but it must be lived forwards.'"

"I'm not sure what that means."

"Neither am I. Most likely those geese over there, see

them? I bet that has never entered their heads either."

"Say, back to the competition thing. The other day I read somewhere about two guys, scientists, who were competing to see who could come up with a vaccine for polio. Both had what it took to make one. But they were at loggerheads as to how it should be taken into the body. One said by needle, the other by spoon. It turned out that, after all the fighting and waste of time and energy squabbling about that in newspapers and so on, both ideas were used. Now doesn't that beat all, that sure seems different than how creatures other than humans get things done."

"Oh, by the way, remember the mystery of the clothes left among the rocks by the lake, making people think a couple of guys swam and drowned? Turns out they didn't. Put a scare in folks though. The two were chased by a gang, wanted the gang to think they had died to get the gang off their backs, to give up the chase. Long time after, the two showed up fit as fiddles, having got out of town."

Ending it All

The plaque on the bench read: *In memory of Sandy Kurushimu.* A man sat staring at the path, green grass, the hard boulders leaning on each other in rows. Then, lifting his tired, bloodshot, tearful eyes, he watched. The waves frothed, spilling over the rocks as water from an overflowing sink. His tears, too, urged him to do something. It had to stop. He felt frightened. So much had gone wrong. So often! He stood, heard a "Good morning," and felt a snuffling mop-faced dog nose his pant leg. No! He hoped the dog wouldn't lift his leg and pee. He felt abused enough.

The warmth of the sun on his head didn't rid him of the cold darkness within as he strode toward the weather-stained bridge. Looking over the rail, he again watched not the unmanageable waves, but some ducks. They lightly bobbed about on the throbbing waves. He watched, stared. A duck's head, then breast, disappeared briefly, mooning him with its rump before surfacing. Ducks always do that. Another duck submerged. Minutes passed. That one maybe gone, a body to mingle with the mud, forever. Then it too popped up, shook itself, and effortlessly bobbed about before sinking out of sight again.

An hour passed, and then two. The black cloud within him moved off. His urge to jump, gag on water, end it all, faded. He felt swimming among the corporate business sharks a possibility, for he, like the ducks, could rise again.

He heard steps on the bridge behind him. A dog's yelp and a voice, loud, nearby, and then the fading "Good day."

"Yes," he whispered. "It's now a good day."

He turned crossed over the bridge and resolved to try again get his personal ducks in line.

His wife must be frantic. He'd been away from home and office for hours. Call his wife. Yes, that's what he will do first, and say "I'm okay now, I'm okay!"

What Makes People Tick?

The two sitting on the park bench kept talking about what makes people do what they do, especially when they think about throwing in the towel.

One repeated that old saying, "When things get tough, the tough gets going."

The other, more of a deep thinker, had his opinions about what motivates people. That motivation word was one he liked. Out came a stream of concepts. He liked the "swim" word too.

"Survival, that's it. People will do anything to survive."

"Okay," said his friend. "But what about the guys who want to end it all?"

"Oh. Sure, there are few exceptions. Territorialism, that's another motivator causing people and animals to get pushy claiming a need for more space.

"That's true," said his friend, "but humans have common sense enough to accept that live and let live is the way to go." "Really?"

What about conflicts? most caused because some want bigger parts of the pie so start wars to hog more land " I can buy into that, I suppose, but I think the bottom line is simply people do what they do because they live between two experiences, pain and pleasure, and the goal is to dissolve or avoid pain, and do anything to seek pleasure.

"Birds and animals, humans the same, but one thing that sets humans apart from other creatures, is humans try to keep from getting bored. Relieving, when you come right down to it, boredom is why people do what they do. Right?"

"Boredom is the feeling everything is a waste of time. Serenity that nothing is."

"Boy, that's heavy!"

His friend, remembering some of his college learning, nodded and added, "Yes, but it's more complicated than that. Humans have four basic needs they have to satisfy, security recognition, response from people, hopefully good strokes, and at least some new adventures to have to tell others about . How does that sound? Does that make sense?"

"Yes, but I've heard it said a little differently."

"Well, there is this guy called Victor Frankl, a psychologist who said that to have meaning in one's life is the ticket. A guy needs something that keeps him going, no matter what. If he doesn't have anything to live for, he won't."

"Suppose that's true," yawned the bench sitter, "but you forget that there are imaginary needs and real needs." He'd learned that from a TV distant learning program.

His friend, not enthralled with that thought, and not knowing how to respond, decided to change the conversation to get at how people connect with each other, thinking that has a lot to do with why people to do the things they, The bench sitter, not wanting to leave any stone unturned, said. "Hold on, you forget people with their heads screwed on right will seek to find their centre. From there they can work on getting their acts together." He had done some pottery and knew if you didn't centre the clay on the wheel, it would go all wonky when you tried to pull it up into a useful shape.

His friend who was sharing the park bench with him said, "It sounds like otherwise, the result would be grotesque, and not be what it was meant to be. Just like in keeping with human's potential."

The bench sitter said, "It sounds like you're getting religious on me. The next thing you're going to say is that humans are spiritual creatures unlike birds and animals."

"That may be so!"

"Well, forget that at least for now. Let's get back to the idea people do what we do to get along with each other. That old book by Dale Somebody or other maybe put a finger on it. *How to Win Friends and Influence People.* Because, you know, each person is not one person but three: the one he thinks he is, the one other people think he is, and the person he really is."

"So what has that got to do with how much tea there is in China?"

"Well, look. A guy has to know how he comes across as a person with others in order to get on track with what he's to do in rubbing shoulders with other people."

"So. We need others to tell us who we are, The next thing

you're going to say is we need others to tell us where to go."

"Look, forget that idea. After all, what it comes down to is this: it's really dog eats dog. The fittest survives. That's what all those survival shows on TV are really about.

We are like mirrors to show us we're not much different than all of nature's other creatures. Just look at any sport. Take hockey for example. Using fancy terms, the game is like life, participation is all pervasive, a social phenomenon. based on elimination by competition, and you can't get away from it. The idea is to be the last standing on top of the hill. Each person needs skill sets to survive. In hockey, it's character, teamwork, and solid work ethics. Same in life. You can say all you want, but what motivates people, makes us tick, is to compete, to survive, and if possible, with the right stuff, to be top dog."

After his friend gave his spiel, his partner sharing the park bench said, "I have heard it said more humanely: be the best that you can be, and remember the ones who succeed are standing on the shoulders of others who made their success possible."

His friend, having the last word, said, "Enough already, you bring tears to my eyes. Let's go have coffee, see what's new."

The Little Boy with a Cardboard Smile

Rutty never smiled. Not only did she not smile, but she did not frown. It didn't matter what she got, a gift, a pleasurable moment, her face remained expressionless. Her loved ones, friends, caregivers tried just about everything to get her to smile. Nothing! Then one afternoon, a visitor brought along a cardboard round happy face with a curved line for a smile. Then he put the face on a stick gave Rutty a candy and laid the face on a table.. All who saw what happened next were astonished. Rutty picked up the smiling face on the stick and held it up to her face. Then Rutty received things, music, whatever would give a "normal" person enjoyment. Rutty greeted these things by holding the smiling stick to her face. But in time, Rutty got tired of smiling that way all the time. The answer? Different round cardboard faces, different expressions, and then Rutty had choices, sad, angry, hurt; thereafter, her blank-faced expression became a way to show how she felt at any time. Like bliss symbols, the face on a stick became a communication tool for those who cannot do so any other way.

*

Somewhere, sometime in another place, a blank-faced boy became a concern. Many tried to get him to respond so he could be a happy, well-adjusted little boy; nothing worked. So, in time, he was thought to be mentally handicapped, his future severely limited. Oh yes, he got simple schoolwork done, did it well, but showed no facial expressions to say, "That was fun," or "too hard," or "easy." He just did it, and when it was done, he did some more.

That was okay till arithmetic became a "can't do."

Kids his age, older, younger, made fun of him. Even he started calling himself a "retard." Then someone, a teacher, parent, friend of the family, read about Rutty a nursing home success enjoyed by a woman who shared her feelings with faces on sticks: happy, sad, more, held up to her blank face, depending on how she felt at any one time. Would this somehow help the little boy, whom others had started to think was hopeless?

That's the way it was, till a grownup gave him a happy face on a stick to hold up to his face when he wanted to show he was happy inside, happy doing schoolwork, happy wherever and whenever. Given arithmetic problems, easy at first, then harder if challenged, he held up the happy face; on and on it went, and to the pleasant surprise of all who knew and cared for him, he wasn't dumb, or dull; he was smart. As his math challenges became harder and his ability to solve easier, he became optimistic. He just needed the happy face mask to accomplish and excel.

But then he ran into a snag. All progress stopped. He had done well challenged by trigonometry problems, but not like he used too. It was no longer easy. Then one day of his struggle and disappointment, by accident, or an inspired moment, a page in a book showed round faces like his happy one, but each had a different expression. By changes of the mouth, drawn down or up, happy could be sad, creases around the eyes could help convey different feelings. Well, the upshot of all that became clear; he was tired of showing he was happy all the time when he wasn't. He could show other feelings he had using other faces on sticks. He wanted to show with the mask more than just his blank, unintentional expression, or his happy one. So, he was given round cardboard faces on sticks showing all kinds of feelings, so he could let others know how he felt on the inside. With that desire fulfilled, he began mastering both trig and calculus, and more. A hopeless little boy no longer, now a genius with a future.

But still, he was lost without his faces on sticks. How to get him to drop those, and with a bold expressive face, be who he was meant to be. He still talked gibberish, withdrew into his blank faced stare. When unmasked he, was still a very unhappy little boy who, without the faces masking his blank exterior, he was lost.

Then again an insightful adult suggested finding a genius to become his friend. The hunt was on, no luck, so few and far between were geniuses. Then, a thought. There was one person known to keep to himself, brilliant, but—he was an old man. Well what was there to lose by getting the little boy genius together with the old one?

The two hit it off. They talked; the boy did so without the round face on a stick, and there was no more gibberish. The two clicked, as friends, colleagues. Thereafter, they were "off to the races." Nothing could stop them—except the old man's death.

Then the question: Would the little genius, now age fourteen, regress or manage progress, or would his achieving continue to depend upon his cardboard masks and gibberish, having him become a one-day wonder? Or would his having connected with the old man set him free "to do his thing" and gain further recognition as a genius, joining the pantheon of the brilliant who perhaps could save the world?

Lots to Live For

Mabel stood at the door of 863 Robinson Street. "Where the hell have you been? I had food ready for you; it got cold, and I threw it in the garbage. What have you been up to, you old fool?" She gave him a kiss on his bald head. "I was about to call the police. You are back, thank God! Why the tears? Why, you're shaking like a leaf! Who is the guy that plunked you down here, he should have put you to bed."

The old man whispered, "That's George, he's my friend, met him after the meeting, he promised to get me home after. I was way over the limit to drive. So George here said he'd get me home in one piece. Thanks, George."

Mabel asked, "But what happened, really, old man, after the meeting? Usually you come home happy, eager to tell me all about being out with your old army pals."

"Don't tell her, George."

"Got too," George said. "You see, it was like this, Mabel.

I was just getting into this guy's car, the one who'd drunk too much to drive. Your old man pulled me aside when I opened the door to climb in and drive him home. He shifted his scrawny bum onto the seat. What could I do? He clung to the steering wheel; nothing would pry him off. So, I didn't take the suicide seat beside him, I sat in the back. The gears made a hell of a noise as he fumbled around, the engine roared. Somehow, we got underway. I asked if he know where he was going. He shouted, 'Damn right! What do think I am? Do you think I don't know my way home?' Turned out he didn't. We ended up going down dark alleys, garbage everywhere, a real nail biter. He cornered so close to the walls, poles scared the hell out me, finally we saw light at an opening to a street—at least at the time that is what I thought it was. He nosed the car's front out, then the rear. *BANG*. Oh my God, I thought we'd had it for sure! Somehow, we both climbed out; this guy who hit us got out. He staggered, leaned on his car's hood, threw up, fell, shouted at us, drunk as a skunk for sure, cursing, 'Your fault! Just look at my beautiful car, it's a write off!'

What did you think your husband did then, Mabel? Why, he looked around, left the car in the middle of the road, stood ram-rod straight at attention in the middle of that street. I shouted, 'For God's sake, get off the road; you'll get killed for sure standing there! He never spoke, just stood like a statue. Cars, trucks veered by him. He just did not budge, what now, call the police? A guy came over, said he's a policeman. I said, 'Okay, you saw what happened.' 'You're damn right I did,' he shouts. 'Well, I ask, "are you going to call it in?" He backed off, looking scared, I said, 'Show me your badge.' He pulled his wallet out, showed me. I say, 'That's a kid's paper sheriff's badge. Get out of here.' 'But I am a witness to the accident! The dunk caused it for sure,' he says.

'Mabel, then another person appeared, I wasn't sure if a man or woman dressed nicely, looked at the car, looked at us, walked around it, almost yawned, no sweat, it's okay, a dent, that's all. But I'll make the call.' After a bit, police arrived, saw your old man looking like he wanted to be killed, so we dragged him to safety, shouting at him, 'You know where you are, this is a highway off ramp.' After a quick inspection of the car, it started okay. Before we left, your husband, needless to say, was not a happy camper. When I climbed into the driver's seat, a police officer said, 'Okay, follow me.' He escorted us to your home, did a U-turn, and was gone, asking no questions. But before he took off, he said little about the cars, more about the drunk driver finishing with, 'You're in the right, that drunk's in the back my cruiser, heading for jail.'

"So Mabel, that's the story."

Mabel says, "Thank God. Fifty years married, did not want to arrange a funeral, prefer a wedding anniversary instead. And as for you, husband. What were you thinking? You don't even have a driver's licence and haven't driven for years!"

George sat beside the old boy, and, like Mabel, asked, "What was all this standing in the middle of the road, daring someone to kill you about?"

The old man looked up from staring at his feet and said, "Nothing to live for, nothing, George, I'm just too tired to go on, want to end it all."

Mabel cried started to cry.

"You will be taken care of Mabel, but I'm useless to you, even in bed. You will find another."

Mabel shouted, "No way."

Then George said, "What about your dog and cat, they'd miss you too. Look, before you do more crazy stuff, get outside, walk around in the park, talk to the ducks; you used to like doing that, feeding the geese. Go meet people again. Your coffee gang, get a life. You deserve that. Mabel needs you, your pets need you, even that stupid turtle you got in the backyard needs you."

Silence, then a whisper, "Okay, I'll give it a try, when I'm sober."

Self-Care in Motion

Spirit Island Park gave those gathered there the chance to share great truths through their actions. Huffing and puffing, hunched over runners, heads-up speeders—who could talk while running—and comfortable joggers passed. Determined, straining, red-in-the-face walkers and casual en-route travellers also circumvented Park Lake. All in motion made a statement, whether conscious of it or not. That harkened back to the ancient Greek philosopher, Halophiles, who said, "When health is absent, wisdom cannot reveal itself, art cannot manifest, strength cannot fight, wealth becomes useless, and intelligence cannot be applied."

Others, lounging on the grass, pronounced another sometimes-neglected truth: "Rest is not idleness, and to lie sometimes on the grass under trees on summer days, listening to the murmur of the water or watching clouds float across the sky, is by no means a waste of time."

Amplifying that observation is the need expressed in a simple, profound way:

"Just living is not enough, one must have sunshine, freedom, and la little flower."

Some persons who found both time and zeal showed they believed it wasn't an either/or decision between leisure or physical exertion on the path, for they showed a believed in doing both.

"True enjoyment comes from activity of the mind and exercise of the body, the two are ever united."

It was true for some. It was all they could do to make it around the park lake while gasping for breath, which verified the idea that "to be or not to be" isn't the question. The question is how to prevent out of breath breathing.

An old spectator offered an alternative to running out of steam while circling the park lake: Adopt the seldom-used scout pace that involved alternating running steps with walking steps. That might help getting around the lake without calling for an ambulance. The Interested old timer observer suggested make eye contact when meeting and passing, to avoid crashing caused by iPhone-addicted.

One other observation that he made did ring a positive note: people spoke many languages as they rounded the lake. He thought, '*How very Canadian!*'

The Prof. and Lone Listener

A professor thought he'd get away and have lunch at the park, sit under a tree, and maybe rehearse his afternoon lecture to the birds. Why not? He found his favourite tree, sat with his back to it, and let his thoughts shuffle into some semblance of order around the topic of loneliness. Since it was a first-year class, he'd keep his lecture simple.

*

Loneliness is a feeling we all experience—especially when a wife, husband or partner dies). Let's think about it, and ways to overcome it. It's been said that Loneliness is nothing new. Artists have expressed feeling lonely. The artist René Magritte, , showed the head of a man and woman about to kiss, but their heads are covered by cloth bags. George Tooker, another painter, showed people in subways lurking about in isolation, staring with fear at each other. Edvard Munch shows people in a death bed scene with backs turned to one another.

Other thinkers speaks of loneliness. Dr. Paul Tournier, Swiss psychologist, claimed, "Loneliness is the most devastating malady of the age." (Tounier 1976). He and others claim, "The rages of loneliness reach deeply into many of our most vexing problems."

Loneliness strikes children of every age, especially those whose parents have little time for them, teens who feel misunderstood and alienated, married couples who feel estranged from their partners, even when living together, and the aged who feel useless and unwanted, even when we have so much to offer.

People can feel alone even when surrounded by others. A poet and novelist, wrote this about loneliness: "Loneliness is most acutely felt with other people, for with others, even with a lover sometimes, we suffer from our differences of taste, temperament, mood" (Sarton 1938)

Another novelist, Faith Baldwin, claimed, "Loneliness can pierce you like a knife on a spring morning or on a golden summer afternoon, no matter where you are or what you are doing. So, who can deny loneliness haunts all." (Baldwin 1964)

The big question is, what causes loneliness? Answer? The deepest cause of loneliness is our human condition itself. Someone said we are born to be alone. Loneliness is not a new human experience. Remember Robinson Crusoe and his longing for a human companion? Author Defoe expressed all our longings for companionship connection and hope found in the person of Robinson Crusoe. Tennessee Williams, in his play *Orpheus Descending,* wrote "We are sentenced to solitary confinement for life in our own lonely skins. We've got to face it, we're under that sentence as long as we live on this earth." (Williams, Orpheus Descending 1958) Why does that have to be? Remember the Bible's Adam who represents humankind? His life illustrates the cause of loneliness, for even when he was united with Eve, he still found themselves out of harmony with his Creator, and thus was still lonely. What impact then does loneliness have upon humans, and how have people tried to deal with it?

There are just too many people that are lonely. Too often loneliness seeps from the pores of our culture. Look at the personal columns of newspaper and magazines often filled with intimate personal ads from people seeking friends or partners. Now the internet is supposed do the trick. Look also at company ads which pick up on this social ailment. One telephoned advertisement read, "Reach out and touch someone"; social media and iPhones serve the same. Real estate firms sell condos advertising us as "Places where you make friends." The lonely feeling is a button for ad-makers to push to get people to buy their answer to loneliness.

Think of all the ineffective ways people try to drain away the feeling of loneliness:

Accumulate Things: Tennessee Williams wrote a play called *The Glass Menagerie.* The play, about escaping reality, has Amanda Wingfield retreating into an illusory world of her youth. I loves her children, but her constant nagging and retelling of her romantic stories are too much for her daughter, Laura. It also drives away her son, Tom. Amanda takes refuge among her glass figurines in the glass menagerie. The figurines become a symbol of her retreat from reality, of loneliness.(Williams, The Glass Menagerie 1945)

Keep Striving: Another way tried to fend of loneliness. In Arthur Miller's *Death of a Salesman:*

Biff: "Are you content Hap? You're a success, aren't you? Happy?"

Hap: "Why no, Biff."

Biff: "Why not, you are making money, aren't you?"

Hap: All I can do now is wait for the merchandise manager to die. And suppose I get to be merchandise manager? He's a good friend of mine, and he just built a terrific estate on Long Island. And he lived there about two months and sold it, and now he's building another one. He can't enjoy it once it's finished. And I know that's just what I'd do. I don't know what the hell I'm workin' for. Sometimes I sit in my apartment—all alone. And I think of the rent I'm paying. And it's crazy. But then, it's what I always wanted. My own apartment, a car, plenty of women, and still, goddamnit, I'm lonely. (Act 1:5 Miller 1949)

A Canadian poet and humourist, when a youth on lonesome nights, finding the hours intolerably long, dialled the long-distance directory assistance from some remote obscure place. Just as bored and lonely, the operator would chat with him about marriage or the weather, pleased for the human contract.

Keep Busy: When single, a young man in an isolated place, not among his own ethnic group, kept busy, thinking he would ward off loneliness as store manager, dispenser of medicine, weather reporter, schoolteacher, and local preacher. But he was terribly lonely.

Feeling sorry for others, thinking we were lonelier than him, a tourist visiting a remote cove, while taking pictures, asked a local, "How can you live so far away from everyone and be so content?" The local answered, "You don't see me rushing to the city to take your picture as you're doing mine, do you?" Anon

What do you think, do any or all of the mentioned ways to stem off loneliness really work?

Having lost to dementia, One lonely ask n asked, why keep on living when your loved one is gone? Especially since in marriage "the two shall become one. But that no longer is true. So what then are the most effective ways to alleviate loneliness, especially when a person is bereaved?

1. Recognize loneliness for what it is, something that sours and sickens the spirit, and something that can't be made a friend. Preoccupation with loneliness is self-poisoning.

2. Learn the difference between loneliness and aloneness. To be alone is neither good nor bad. How I use my time of solitude will determine if it is good or bad. A widower cried, "Being alone so colours one's life." Another widower replied, "But isn't it nice to choose your colour?"

3. Remember it's okay to be alone. It is often necessary to be alone to create. Everyone needs periods of aloneness to reflect on what's been done.

4. Try creativity to help you get through the loss of a loved one or friend, and to reconnect with nature and others.

An author found that he was running dry. He couldn't think what to write. He had lost his gift. He couldn't function. He felt as though he was having a nervous breakdown. He visited his doctor for a prescription. The doctor told him to go to Spirit Park Lake and open four envelopes, one every three hours.

At nine a.m., he opened the first. The note said, *Listen.* For three hours he listened to the water, the birds, the people. He listened to sounds that he hadn't heard for years.

At twelve noon, he opened the second envelope. *Try to reach back*, the note said. For three hours he tapped his memory about where he and his wife had been and what they had done with their lives together.

At three, he opened the third envelope: *Remember your original motives*, it said, for three hours the author asked himself, *why did I start? Would I do it again? Why did I do it? Say that? React that way?*

At six, the author opened the last envelope. It said, *Write your worries and fears*. For three hours he put his resentments, worries, and fears on paper, then he burned it. That's creative solitude. Anon

It's been said, "We are called to be alone together, not so private that we do not miss our responsibilities, nor so work-orientated that we miss solitude." Someone else piped up, "The way to deal with loneliness is to learn about risk-takers' lives. By doing so, you may find you can take a strong stand on something, running against the stream, and find that even alone you risked and survived."

Involve yourself in service. Seldom can a person be lonely that way. Find a family-like community. The claimed Community is the best answer to the universal sense of loneliness in this life (Colleagues 2001)

*

The professor, rising from the grass, brushed himself off, and hoping his lecture wouldn't just be for the birds, moved across the grass toward his car. Still, he didn't notice the silent lone figure leave his outdoor lecture hall and walk by himself, down the path, his head down, and hands shoved deep in his pockets. No one else seemed to notice him either.

Talk about Happiness

Two middle-aged women, experienced empty nests; their children had flown the coop.

One, sighing wistfully, said, "The kids made me happy, at least most of the time. Now what?"

The other, a real gung-ho, outdoorsy type said, "Happiness, you know, has a whole lot to do with getting in touch with oneself in relationship with nature. Take this Spirit Park for example, I once read 'Happiness is one long continuous chain of little joys, little whispers from nature, little rays of sunshine's daily work.'"

"That sounds a bit soppy!"

"Yes, I guess, maybe, but heck Anyway, you can have lot of fun, whether it's in the park or in the home, even when you don't know you are having it."

"I read about a three year old helping her mom bake a cake. Mom stirred while the girl added dates and eggs to the mixture. As she was about to add the vanilla, she looked up at her mom with a grin and whispered glee-fully, "Are we making a mess?"'

Her friend, swallowing the story, said, "Oh, stop, now you are reminding me of my kids again, and the home stuff."

"Okay, then look at it this way. You see that person ahead of us being pushed in a wheelchair?"

"So?"

"Well, when I taught school, I shared stories with the kids about the idea you don't need to rely on circum-stances to make you happy. I remember the story about Lord Byron and Sir Walter Scott: Both were lame. Byron was downright miserable with his lameness. He brooded on it till he loathed it. He never entered a public place, and sure not a park. For him, he didn't see any way he could get any more buzz out of life. Much of the zest of living was gone.

"Scott, on the other hand, never complained. He never spoke a bad word about his disability, not even to his closest friend. It's not surprising one day Scott got a letter from Byron that concluded, "Scott, I would trade my fame to have your happiness."

"Well, thanks for that. It's a good story. But what about us? We're not the kind that will be remembered, like those two big guys." "Okay, maybe we're not the heavy-weights of society."

"Stop right there, and that's another thing, trying to

be happy and lose weight at the same time doesn't make one happy."

"I'm not talking about that. I'm remembering someone else, don't know if he had a weight problem or not, or if he could make it around the park without gasping for air; I'm remembering Louis May Alcott, who wrote at age twelve in her diary, "Had good dreams and woke now and then to think and watch the moon; I had a pleasant time with my mind, for it was happy.'"

"See, there you are, it doesn't take much to make a person happy. We can be happy right here, in the park. Sure, there is no moon out, though I saw a faint glimpse of one early this morning, but you and I have lots of good stuff to think about, the grass, birds, trees, a whole lot of stuff around us to enjoy. "Let's get with it."

Her friend, not totally convinced, turned and said, "Just like that, eh, so simple. I'm not convinced. Even though I'm in the park where everything seems so fresh and vibrant , reflections in the water today looking like glass, such doesn't mirror them. Why does it take so much convincing to get persons to realize that they don't have to feel we need to remain eternally young to be happy? Look at that guy over there, the one with the paunch wearing sweats. It's just like a man to see that he does not need to protest that he's not over the hill."

"Yes, that's true. Somewhere in one of my movie magazines, I read about one actor who said, "I may not have lived wisely, industriously, virtuously, but I have lived happily. I am not an introspective man, but I am, I hope a grateful one. Life has left me kindly, and should I suddenly withdraw her favours, I hope I shall always be mindful that over fifty years the sun shone on by back."

"Sounds a bit corny."

"Maybe, but it can't be any more maudlin than this bit I read in some self-improvement book—I can't remember which one. I think I've just about read them all."

"Who, then, are the happy ones?

"The happy are the ones who know how to live with the unknown without feeling threatened or frightened. The happy are those who accept the unknown—even seek the unknown. Being willing to face the unknown allows one to meet a wide variety of people easily and naturally regardless of age, education, class, or colour. The happy are those who know that there is no adventure without uncertainty. The happy are the grateful. The happy are those who appreciate again and again the basic goods of life, however, others may think otherwise."

Her friend responded, "You know that culvert that we were digging up the other day? Well, when I jogged by the guys digging around there, I thought of one of my profs. I think he's dead now, but he said there was this economist. He was watching a workman digging a ditch. He looked at how the dirt kept the shape of the shovel as it flew through the air and landed exactly where the workman wanted it. Like an apprentice approaching his master, the economist joined the workman and practised shovelling until he had learned the knack of it."

"Okay, I got the drift of that, but are there any more of your goodies, the happy stuff?"

"Yes, a couple more. Do you like them?"

"What's to like. I just thought that you were happy spieling them off. I didn't want to spoil your fun."

"Well, if that's the little you're getting from me, I'll stop right there."

"No, please go on, you've got my attention. I'm with you."

"Let's think what makes a person happy. The happy are people with a mission in life who aren't self-centred. Happiness for me is the by-product of work and duty. Maybe this is the reason mothers with babies seldom get sick, unlike others. The happy are also realists who can detect fake, dishonest."

Her friend interrupted, "Hey, don't we go through life wearing rose-coloured glasses or through glass darkly?"

"That's not the point; see what is there rather than own, hopes, and fears. don't complain about water because it's too wet, or rocks because are too hard, or a competitor because she beat you in a contract. See people as they really are, and thus be seldom disappointed in others. The happy don't blink at ills and injustices around them, but neither do they believe the world can be set right overnight through social and political panaceas.

Happy people like to do useful, productive work, to use their abilities fully to enjoy helping people. But are not doormats! They tend to be self-sufficient and enjoy both solitude and company but aren't dependent on either. Happy persons dislike cruelty and destructiveness, healthy persons have no hang-ups about prosperity and refuse to participate in other people's negative emotions or cling to their own."

"Where did you get that list from?"

"I can't remember. I've read a lot of stuff. I also remember reading about a pilot—"

"And what was that about?"

"There was this pilot trapped in the desert for two days. He found an orange in his plane wreck. Stretched out beside a fire, he looked at the orange and said to himself that men didn't know what an orange was. He who was condemned to die, thought to himself. Still that certainty couldn't compare with the pleasure he was feeling. The joy he took from the pleasure he was feeling of holding that orange in his hand. That was one of the greatest joys he had ever known." Anon

"Isn't that something?"

"So, what you are saying, and what it all comes down to is, thank God for small mercies."

"Bertrand Russell claimed to be without some things you want are an indispensable part of happiness. See I read, too!"

"Hurrah for you! I think you got it. I don't know what movie star it was. But she said, I think it was her, 'We're made for enjoyment and the world is filled with things that we can enjoy, unless we are too proud to be pleased with them, or too grasping to care for what we receive."

"I guess that's something like what I found in a book called *The River* by R. Goodens. One person in the book asked the other, 'How can I be happy?' Her friend answered, "It isn't for us to dictate. If you are happy, you are. You can't make yourself happy"

"We're part of something greater than ourselves. That's what I read. I guess it's something like being part of Spirit Lake Park, do you think?"

"I guess that's true. Just try to tell my perfectionist, self-made ex-husband about it. My clergy friend a few Sundays back quoted from a guy called Gerald Kennedy: 'A young married man read many the psychoanalysis and religious self-help books on how to adjust to life, marriage, and to other difficulties. His young wife, who tried to live up to the precepts in these books, one day rebelled: 'Now that we've found real happiness. Couldn't we now have some fun?'

"It sounds somehow as if she got a raw deal, if she thought deprived,"

I'm getting in the zone, like a hockey goalie."

"You like hockey? Never mind. Now, since we split, I'm like the lady in Thornton Wilder's play, *Our Town*. (Wilder

1938) This person did get a second chance. She died. But was given the opportunity to re-live one day of her life. She got more out of that day of course, experiencing human existence for the second time for she saw how marvellous it was being alive. I guess, like that person, I'm noticing in the park and in other places so much free stuff, to see and take in, to be happy.

So happiness, as one poet said, is made up of minute fractions—the little, soon forgotten, the sight of two children sitting on a log talking and eating apples. The smell of pine gum warming in the bright afternoon sun."

"Just look around you, right?"

"Right!"

The Teacher's Discovery

She stood, fingers spread on the sweaty, sticky cover of the new biology text while staring at the windowless walls and remembering the spruce-scented air, and the lake's freedom-loving breeze. School halls and classrooms had a heavy smell, tainted by pungent loose-laced runners, so expensive, the latest styles, yet so boring. With her hair tossed back in the breeze, arms swung wide, elated, she had danced through summer, and now gazed at the wall clock. It shared the light of the cold fluorescence shining on baseball-cap-headed boys and on bare-bellied girls.

Thinking she, too, needed a gradual sinking into the seats for another heavy semester, heard herself say,

"Class. as planned, we are going over to the park to gather water specimens for this semester." She glanced around the class, trying to break up the clique scrums and rouse the sleepy singles with her voice and eyes.

For a moment the thought took the shape of a picture, the park's lake giving urine-like specimens to the clinically trained. The idea of breaking out of a dry-walled classroom got the desks scraping, feet shuffling; there was a scramble for the door.

"Hold on," she said, "pick up jars and dip nets, I'll meet you at the dock."

Walking towards the dock, this teacher thought of the reflective time she enjoyed that summer at the cottage by another lake, one where haunting loon calls echoed off the surrounding hills. There, often sitting on the end of the dock, paddling bare feet in the cool, clear water, and brushing away pesky mosquitoes and flies. Every year with her escape from the classroom came encounters, not only with pesky insects, but with persistent thoughts for urgent attention. Biological dissecting of the bodies of frogs that resembled human physiology, though visceral, was a snap compared to dissecting one's thoughts to reveal haunting conundrums common to her and her colleagues' concerns.

Without fail, problems kept her summer from pure, earthy joy. It drove her to seriously reflecting on life while often alone. Her weekend visitors returning to city jobs, left her talking out loud, having one-way conversation with nature's living things begging squirrels and sheltering trees. Her thoughts transformed into words mingling with other sounds drifting down from the canopy of green above her shake-roofed cottage, its front yard a sandy beach. Like Spirit Island Park had power to lift one's dusty mouldy memories or unresolved issues off lives, so also did her creature-comfort sanctuary do the same.

Like stuff hidden and neglected in a fridge drawer or cupboard, every summer, these items whispered, "Do you want to keep us, or pitch such from her mind?" and every summer she tried again to clear her head, unclutter her mind to invade the minds of the latest versions of the hormone-driven and zit-concerned students. Only human creatures could give up indulging in self-consciousness and self-doubt. True, there are other things kept lingering in minds that humans could easily do without.

When I get back at it in September, she mused, *there will be a new horde of kids invading my lab and my seat of emotions, a bunch tormented within by feelings of envy, brains not yet able to settle self-images as being okay.*

Throughout her thought journey, nature's orchestra, birds, frogs, and insects, supported her in the ongoing sorting process. In her apartment, she shoves a CD into the player, but no sounds matched those of nature. Even the faint thundering and lightning, beginning to give legitimacy to the dark, bloated clouds moving into her visual space, helped compress her thoughts into oozing, fruitful ideas to work through.

How, when she got back to school, could she convince the teens to risk a little more, to give up peer acceptance security blankets and begin to grow out of their awkwardness? Perhaps, where and if success surfaced would it help by supplying students with images? Such as the *Peanuts* cartoon's Linus dragging around his security blanket woven from poor self-esteem? Would they retain the message? As their teacher urging to think about how we humans, as nature's other creatures, may be so self-conscious and worried to death with an inferiority complex, that we can't focus on what we are meant to do to reach full potential as human beings. When she arrived back from holidays determined to try again to escape from lethargy? To do that, she would have to share the futility of envying others. I would tell the story of singer Buffy St. Marie's discovery. Buffy used her voice, personality, and money to help her Indigenous people. Buffy once told that her first ambition was to be a cheerleader, then an airline stewardess, like the average girl. But as an average girl, she failed. So, she decided to be herself.

With that message of Buffy's, the teacher thought that what she'd do differently would encourage her students to keep their minds be less distracted by self-doubt and fear of rejection, to keep o open the indoors of their minds to focus outwardly enjoying nature's gifts of sun and rain.

How, I asked herself, could she inject a breath of fresh air into the minds of those kids who felt rejected by their peers, who dumped doubts and fears on them through snide remarks and cruel ganging up? How would she get across to the lonesome abused that it is not their fault they suffer put downs. It's all instigated by insecure abusers with hang-ups of their own.

How could she reach the down-and-outers, convincing them worth is not dependent on others?

One colleague of hers, a high school drama teacher, once told her a truth to pass on to her students. He said, "No one can take the role of playwright and stage manager in our lives. We should not depend on others to give us worth."

Having received that past-it-on truth, she reflected on her summer holiday experiences. "As I'd sat bailing water out of my boat at the cottage after a cloud burst," she told her colleague "I thought it incredible that certain bits of what I read—beyond the actual professional material— often sufficed to fill my consciousness with useful concepts to share with my students. I thought of the time I'd spent away from the city, alone, stock-taking of my life.

I remembered an exercise one of my own teachers had the class do; each student took a piece of paper and listed his or her good points. One of her students put up her hand and asked, "Teacher, can I use both sides of the paper?"

That remembrance felt good, but in my years of teaching, I'd come to the conclusion, as many teachers had, that unless some students can clear their minds of feeling like real clumsy klutzes, they would never have sufficient healthy empty space in their thoughts to learn."

Her flashbacks to her summer at the cottage ended abruptly. Her feet found her way down the path to the pier. She hadn't realized how she had dawdled. All her students were already there, by Spirit Lake, their bodies lounging on grass, some leaning over water, some nudging and pushing while young eyes, teeth, and mouths shaped an array of feelings—some bored others eager, some confused. Now that their leader had arrived, they became cool, nonchalant, drifting over to where she stood with her clipboard rattling off instructions, motivated by tried-and-tested verbal tricks to rouse the troops to action. "The goal: fill the jars with scummy water, visually inspect the contents for signs of life, record your findings, share those with others, after half an hour, meet me back at the lab."

Off they went, some looking like bear cubs swatting the water for fish, some like awkward, young deer, cautiously and vigilantly dipping r graceful necks to sample the water.

The teacher was about to head back to the school. I abruptly stopped fantasizing and mumbled to her, *Not likely, cubs or fawns!* Then she watched and listened to the chatter, shouts, and laughter. All seemed to be moving about in clumps—all except one lean, awkward youngster who held back, balancing on the rocks, seemingly absentmindedly poking away at the water with the wooden-handled dip net. The others paid no attention to him. She began walking toward him. He either didn't seem aware of her approaching, or didn't care.

"What did you find, Louis?

"Lou," she whispered.

"Oh, yes, Lou. Anything interesting?"

"I don't know what to do," he spat out between almost closed lips, briefly glancing her way.

His grey, peaked face, tired eyes and faded straw-coloured hair down around his ears triggered empathy. More so , his teasing the collar of a well-worn jacket softened what his teacher was about to say next.

She remembered some of what she'd recalled during the summer at the cottage, inviting Lou over to sit with her on a bench nearby. Seated, she said, "Forget the dip net, Let's talk." she didn't try to pry out of him what was bugging him. His distance from the group made that perfectly clear. She didn't feel bad when his awkwardness muzzled his mouth from sharing the obvious pent-up feelings of worthlessness and smouldering hurt. As his teacher she knew a little about this boy from school records, and from other teachers.

So I talked softly. He appeared to listen willingly.

"Lou, I knew a teacher once who asked one of her young pupils, 'What was the most valuable invention in the world?' You know what he answered?"

"Don't know."

"The little guy shouted, 'Me!'"

Lou leaned over, peered down at his ragged runners with knotted laces, and said, "How can he say that?"

"Lou, you can say that too."

"No!"

"Yes, because you, me, we, are all valued that way, even when we sometimes don't think so."

He rubbed one foot over the other, still staring down, and whispered, "I don't think so."

"Well, it's true, Lou. Believe it. You know, I heard some-where, and I believe it to be true, that what gives a person worth is not what others think of him but the cause that he identifies with. If the cause is trivial, merely self-serving, then, it will not be surprising if that person thinks poorly about himself. There is an old expression, 'Hitch your wagon to a star.' Maybe you had a grandmother who said that. It still holds true."

"I don't got a grandma, but I got an uncle who played hockey. Good at it too!"

"What did you hear him say about all we've talked about?"

"He didn't"

"How come, Lou?"

"He's dead, shot himself."

Before she heard that, she had planned to go on, saying, "It's sad that some people, driven by our own feelings of inadequacy, will go to great lengths to achieve. We often fail, not because we do not have worth, but because we have chosen the wrong vocation, calling, or venture, a square peg in a round hole. It's also sad society rewards high performing athletes with big bucks, expecting us to be to be miracle workers, often driving us to the point of exhaustion. But it is wonderful, people will give others the opportunity to fail and learn from our mistakes, even trust us with very important responsibilities."

My God, I thought, *what am I thinking anyway!*

Lou straightened up, turned, touched her shoulder lightly, looked up into her eyes, glistening with a film of tears, and got up to leave. Then his lips shaped gentle words: "It's okay."

Hugs Are Miracles Too

One was a crusty grey-moustached man, obviously the father of the other, a slim, fast walker. They looked about, commenting back and forth as they rounded the lake.

The older one pointed to a pathetic-looking gander; appearing tired and arthritic, barely making it over the rocks and on to the grass. "You see that? Not much hope he'll be joining the flock heading south this fall. Don't think I'll be making it either. It'll be a miracle if I even make it through the winter. Damn prostate!"

"You never know," the younger said. "Miracles do happen."

The old man coughed. "Seems the only time a miracle happens is when someone wins the 649 lottery."

"Oh, I don't know about that. I think it just depends on how you define a miracle."

"Getting academic on me son, next thing you know you're going to use big words again.

"Maybe big thoughts, but big words, no. I don't think I believe that a miracle takes place once in a blue moon. When something very extraordinary seldom happens, but when it does it is to a very special few a miracle, the odds being a million to one."

"Well," said the older man, coughing again, "that cuts me out, I ain't no special person."

"To me, you are. Sometimes miracles happen all around us throughout our lives and cannot be considered trivial. Birth, that's a miracle. Our very lives are fragile miracles, recovery from an illness is a miracle, the changing of a life is a miracle."

"Yeah, okay, but just suppose I don't beat the crappy cancer, does that mean no miracle for me?"

"Look, sometimes, you know, the miracle for us is something altogether different from what we wanted."

"Well that's fine, son. I guess I can live with that least as long as I'm around."

"I heard it kicked around the table down at Timmy's about miracles. As some guys put it, one's that we all can be thankful for health." His son, feeling his dad warming up to the idea that miracles do happen, dumped the whole bale of ideas on the old man. "Dad, modern equipment with sophisticated innards and fine-tuned engineering is still vulnerable to breakdown. It's a miracle our bodies are so much more complex than the most intricate human-devised equipment, do as well we do. That's a miracle isn't it?

The father lifted himself painfully from the park bench, shuffled over the rocks lining the lake. He stared bleary-eyed at some geese with goslings and,, with his back to his son, rasped, "I suppose they, too, miracles like us. You think, son?"

"Sure, Dad, come on and sit back down. Now as I was saying"

"Would you say that fly buzzing around my head bugging me, that's a miracle, too?"

"Yes, Dad, that too, but just as I was about to tell you— listen, Dad, the point to consider is this: We as a people have advanced. But have we advanced so far that we can legitimately dismiss the evidence of miracles? Isn't it true we know less and understand less, more and more?"

"Son, can you reach down and pick up that feather there? I wonder what bird that came from. Would you know? Kind of like the Creator's writing instrument, do you think?"

"A bit far-fetched, Dad. Now getting back to what I was explaining to you. Science has performed miracles in keeping people alive longer. Penicillin has saved many. Antibiotics have and vaccines have rescued even more from dreadful diseases. People who wear glasses survive. Would many of us have survived back then if physically handicapped, or short sighted, as we do now? Not likely! But has all this improved the quality of life for those who live longer?"

"Do you want me to answer that?"

"No, that's okay. Let's get on with what I was saying. But of course, scientists have not lost faith in the idea miracles can and will occur. We still believe that the impossible is going to happen. And the incredible that's predicted will often turn out to be true. For instance, the sun, astronomers say, is cooling off, burning itself out, and millions or billions of years from today it will die, leaving the earth with no heat or light. People, we say, will either crawl deep into the bowels of the earth, closer to the raging heat of the earth's core, or we will move to another habitable planet, if such exists."

The dad, oblivious to his son's words, peered out at the weed-woven surface of the water, and said, "You know, son, my body will soon be part of the mud for water plants to grow in this lake. You did agree to scatter my ashes here, right?"

His son gave him a pained look and continued, "You

know, our very existence on this planet is a miracle of the greatest proportions. What do you think about that?"

The dad turned, peered into his son's face intently through bleary, tired eyes, and it was in that moment his son realized that his dad, who had been his parent, his teacher, had now given that role over to him. His dad . . . DID NOT HAVE HIS HEARING AIDS ON!

"Dad," the son shouted. "You tired? Want to walk some more, maybe talk some more before we head back to the lodge? Or do you want to just sit right here?"

"Sure, okay, what were you talking about again?"

"Miracles, Dad, different kinds. You know, across the centuries, many deserts have been changed into productive places. Miracles! I heard somewhere about a person, one of many, who, after an ear operation, cried out, 'Doctor, I can hear!' The doctor had replaced the smallest bone in the human body with a wisp of stainless steel, a wire implant, a miniaturization, a miracle. Wow! Right, Dad?

"But even a greater miracle yet, most have heard about this one. You have!"

Silence. His dad must have been listening intently; he had put his hearing aids on.

"Dad, so what do you think of that? Dad? Dad! You've fallen asleep. I'm sorry! What can I do for you?"

"Huh? Oh. You can give me a hug, son. I like hugs."

The Bike and Marked Bills

Shuffling along around the lake, he stopped by the park bench near the pavilion, downwind of the dock. He lifted one leg, bent his knee, pressed his runner on the lip of the park bench and leaned over, pulling his right shoelaces in to tie a tighter knot. Annoyed at having to stop, he indulged himself, as he often did, by analyzing the why of it.

Without fail, he blamed it on his right foot, smaller than his left, and his right leg bowed a bit, causing that foot to go along with the leg, pulling unevenly on the lace. He laboured in his head the cause of his annoyance, one of the many he encountered on his trips around the park's lake. In each instance he dug around in his memory for answers to the causes of his inconveniences. Not only did he do that, but he contended with the unexpected.

Gee. He stopped cold. *See that guy, almost hit me a side blow with his bike. Sometimes it's better to keep walking or running. A moving target is harder to hit! Laces tied up, head up like a hockey player, no good having your head down stick handling, you're just welcoming a hard hit, same if you're deep in thought trying to untie knotty problems.*

It seemed unless a person got off the path, he was fair game for single-minded bike riders or by other speeders aided by human devices. When fast bike peddlers, in-line skaters, or skateboarders charged up without warning, the startled walker had a split second to decide whether the threat would pass on the left or right. A guy gets the message a person needs be on his toes when sharing the path, even in supposedly tranquil park setting. You just never know when something will unexpectedly come at you out of the blue. "Stay alert or you'll get hurt," ought to be the motto of fast-paced livers who invade nature's sanctuary. In contrast, the ones with the persistent dragging shoelaces have discovered some people remain oblivious to the park's tranquility.

Off the beaten path, among the trees, some gathered around a picnic table drinking tea. The smell of bannock and meat cooking on a charcoal barbecue pleasantly scented the air, taming the stench of rotting weeds sliming the surface of the lake, near the dock. Laughing, climbing, wrestling, rough-housing teens, infants, toddlers, mothers, and dads. If snapshotted, one would catch a moment where a few native families, used to rural reserve life, enjoyed a respite from the concrete sterility and indifference of the city.

Shadows of approaching evening settled on the trees that created nature's canopied green leafed dome. Voices of families, elders, replaced the chorus of joking, kibitzing with tales of gritty living, spiked often with unexpected endings. One story began and soon caught and held the attention of the drooping-eyed youth who, intrigued, began to listen intently.

"Remember when the coal miners laboured underground and lived good and bad times in this city? I was about then with a handful of friends who hadn't found a place on the reserve. So we worked in the States, did a lot of overtime and crossed back over the border into Canada with a fat roll of money, twenty thousand dollars to be exact. We were so darn happy that we even treated ourselves to a stay in a motel instead of sleeping in our rickety fume-filled van. The only thing as good was the new decoration on the van's top, a brand new bike for a kid brother back on the reserve—a promise made, soon to be fulfilled.

"Two days later, the dream and some others came crashing down. The friends were hauled out of our beds by ski-masked motel home-invaders. The intruders knew what they were after. They roughed up one friend, who was forced to give them all the money he was carrying for us. All but the very little spent disappeared out the door, gone within minutes, followed by the roar of a hot truck engine."

The storyteller, no doubt, must have been one of the unfortunate friends. For he dramatized his tale with first-hand conversation. He said, "You know it was just like it was yesterday. I can remember just about every word of our conversation about that whole business."

"That was hell," one shouted.

"You are telling me!"

"Worse than that, all that hard work for nothing," cried another.

"Heck, just when we think we're doing the right thing, telling welfare what they can do, we're back to square one," a third piped in.

The last friend, who had been very quiet, finally bellowed, "It's worse than that. We got that whacking big motel bill, no credit card, and that beat up gas guzzler out there, no telling if we wanted to make a quick getaway without paying the bill, or if that rust-bucket van would even get us far. Besides, who wants that hassle anyway?"

The friends, down in the mouth, had sprawled around the motel room, looking like death warmed up. Silence and gloom filled the room, suddenly broken by one who had been pacing back and forth swearing under her breath. She stopped; a faint smile formed on her tired face. The defeated look washed away, leaving a brighter, eye-sparkling appearance. Each of her friends sat up. "What? What gives? What are you looking so silly about? This is no laughing matter."

"Maybe not, but then again," she answered, "I remember something. There was this guy in the restaurant, the table across from us, he looked pretty interested in our roll of cash. I peeled off some to pay the bill. I heard his name. His friend used it when they talked together. I got the idea he and his buddy worked in the mine. Name's Keelo. I remember that because it was so different."

"So, how's that going to help?" asked her friend, his elbow propped up beside her.

"So we tell the police that it's Keelo who ripped us off.

"Then what? Even if he still got the money, and the police get it from him, or from his buddy, how is that going to help us? How can we prove the money is ours?"

"Well, I just thought of something I did when I first got charge of the money from you guys. I didn't tell you what I did . You might have poked fun at me."

"So, what did you do?" A couple of us laughed.

"You might not believe it, but, well, I printed each bill with my mascara."

"You think that will do the trick and get our money back?" one chuckled. "That would be one up on that white guy Keelo, if he's the rip-off artist."

"Worth a try. Let's get the police on board. Phone our own RCMP on the reserve. Don't know the ones here. And in the meantime, while he gets his act together, let's check the local thrift shop. Need a bike for my little guy back home. Got a few bucks left. Maybe get one to replace the new one stolen off top of the van," said the oldest of the friends, who looked a little more with it, less pessimistic.

The storyteller was now getting to the good part. His look got listeners eager for more. He chuckled, "I should have been onstage, eh? Quite a performance from an old fart like me."

Anyway, what happened was this.

The RCMP got our man. He did it, and because the smart lady among us men had ID'd the money, we got most of it back. By the way, we got one rusty bike from the thrift shop before hearing the good news. We fixed it up using the tools from the van, and some bit of paint and stuff. Sold it, bought a better one, and you can believe it or not, bought a couple more! Piled them on the van roof, exhaust-fumed it back to the reserve. There's more! A couple of us characters, once down in the mouth, who had been ripped off, thought we'd buy, fix up, and sell bikes. We did, and we had so much fun doing it. If you drive down the main drag on the reserve, you'll see a sign reading "COMMUNITY BIKE STORE: Get your bikes here, cheap."

That's some story!

"But that's not the end of it," said the storyteller. "There is this guy—looks like Santa Claus. Call him the 'Bike Man.' Lives off the reserve in another town. He collected antique bikes—even had one manufactured by John Deere. We, reserve bike store owners bought his collection. If we hadn't, it most likely would have just rusted away. It seemed Bike Man's town hadn't shown interest in helping preserve and display his bikes. But his efforts didn't fall by the wayside. The bike store and museum on the reserve became something to behold, visited by many who found evidence that "We can do this" had become "We did it!"

Now We See Dimly, as in a Dark Mirror

Two high school friends, Mark and Beth, cut through Spirit Lake Park on their way to and from school most days. Their talk on route centred on the usual interests and troubles common to their peers. Shakespeare's *Hamlet* also kept cropping up in conversations, seemingly uninvited—partly because it was required reading that semester, and even more so because of that "to be or not to be" quote. It haunted their thoughts, where the big questions of life roamed around begging answers.

The two became very familiar with the park's natural furniture, so much so that only new additions would have had a chance of getting their attention, so preoccupied were they with teen concerns. During high school years, using the park for a shortcut, they noticed, and quickly shrugged off, dismissing from our minds, weird characters who appeared and, in time, disappeared, but one Friday afternoon on the way home, they both heard something strange, a sound that just didn't blend in or contribute to the chatter they had become accustomed to in the park. It came from a fragile-looking, grey-haired woman who appeared to be reading out loud to her dog. The teens casually moved closer, hoping the woman wouldn't be distracted and stop reading. She wasn't and didn't. We listened and heard: "'Hannah.' Paul's voice sounded remote and spent, yet the tone predicted an important announcement.

"Hannah, I've done a great deal of thinking tonight, emergency thinking. I've never taken much interest in the idea that the things we do, and the things we believe, can influence, in any way, whatever powers there may be outside and beyond ourselves, and I'm not sure even now that I have faith to offer. My mind is upset, and I know I'm not using it according to its habits. But so many people have believed and do believe. I've been groping about to see if I could do it too. I've even tried to pray. But that seems a hypocritical thing for me to do."

The two teens soon nodded to each other having heard enough and continued on their way, barely mentioning what they'd heard

On Monday afternoon, to their surprise, the same woman sat reading to her dog, In the weeks that followed, the woman whom they had written off as just another eccentric—often frequented the same bench, reading aloud. Many more weeks passed with no change. Finally, the teens just had to satisfy our curiosity. They just had to find out something, anything, about the strange person who had become more than merely a park novelty, but a fixture. So one late afternoon, the two sidled over to her bench, sat down, and, staring at the lake, small talked their way into feeling more comfortable with her.

To their surprise, she wasn't mad. In fact, she seemed quite normal for an old person.

After we had left the woman and her dog—Plato—and started home, those teens noted that if anything, their new acquaintance had a charismatic personality.

"Certainly not one like the witch that enticed juicy children into her gingerbread house," Beth said.

"Whatever were you thinking," Mark laughed.

"I don't know just kids' stuff."

"You and I aren't kids anymore. In fact, we should be able to talk to this person. She seems to make sense. For fun, let's ask her about *Hamlet*'s, 'to be or not to be'—that's one of life's big questions right?"

So the next week, they conversed with the interesting woman. It soon led to surprise—an unpacking that big question and the whole business about beliefs, especially about a belief in a Creator, or "Higher Power."

The two found their acquaintance becoming a credible friend. Her name was Priscilla. She was a retired philosophy professor nd found the park a comfortable place to reflect and enjoy the company of anyone interested in visiting with her and her dog, Plato.

Persons happening to listen in on the three conversing would hear stimulating questions and answers that continued for several weeks.

Priscilla found the girl and boy intelligent and interested in the big questions of life. So she began to enjoy their questions and the opportunity to respond, letting the two take the lead in bringing up concerns they had about what they did or didn't believe.

Mark cautiously mentioned guys he knew who talked about such stuff but weren't sure what to believe, or really didn't care.

Priscilla said, "That sounds familiar. I went through

that bit. I didn't know what I believed. Someone once said this, which is about where I was at in my thinking long ago, 'I might be described as a tourist in the religions landscape.' Once the whole business was very confusing for me. I even felt some people were telling me I should believe in this or that. I was hearing from people who were well-versed in religious thought. But rather than convince me of anything, they actually did the opposite.

"I wasn't the only one who felt that way. I read once about an incident where a minister thought he had preached well on atheism. After, he asked the farmer what he thought of his sermon.

"'Well,' the farmer said, 'you spoke a lot, and no doubt that was very clever, but I still believe there is a God.'

Beth asked, "Priscilla, do you believe in God too?"

Priscilla answered, "Yes, it would be harder not to."

"How so?" Beth looked puzzled.

Priscilla said, "I once had a student who, like many others, scoffed at the idea of believing in a God. He even went further saying, 'I think when you're dead, you're dead, and that's all there is to it.' I said, 'Then you're an atheist.' He said, 'No, I don't believe in that either.'"

"Now, that's weird," Mark said.

"That's right, it is, but that way of thinking is common among both atheists and agnostics."

"Agnostics?" Mark asked,

Priscilla explained. "People called agnostics aren't sure

if there is a God. Then there are the atheists. Many have said unfair things, for instance: 'An atheist is a person who has no invisible means of support.' Or, 'An atheist is one who wish to God he could believe in God.'

Or, lastly, 'The atheist is one who tries to pull God from his/her throne, and set up instead the phantom chance.'"

Beth said, "I'm not sure if those glib, negative comments throw much light on the issue at hand!"

Priscilla said, "You are correct, it doesn't! Let's look at it differently: To be an atheist, you need to have more faith in believing in nothing than what it takes to believe in a God. Also, try giving up believing. You'll find there is no acceptable alternative, for you can't believe against something. You can only believe in it. So, you see, it doesn't make sense to say, 'I don't believe in God.' Now, if you want to sit on the fence and say, 'I do believe there may be a God, I'm just not sure,' then you've caught yourself in a bind. For to say that I am an agnostic is a contradiction. Why? Because we all believe in something. Emptiness remains only for a moment and no longer.

"One day a person bumps into a friend who is a believer. Her friend asks, 'Is it true you no longer believe?'

"Her friend answers, 'God forgive me, I'm now an atheist.'

"The fact that I includes God in this way indicates I must still believe in the existence of God. What's wrong with an atheist's line of reasoning can be summed up in this statement: 'An atheist cannot find God for the same reason a thief cannot find a policeman.'

"One other problem atheists, and even agnostics, have is this: We are so preoccupied with looking in the most unlikely places to find truth. It's so easy to limit one's view of the world.

"One poet put it this way: 'The world is not a prison house, but a kind of spiritual kindergarten where millions of bewildered infants are trying to spell God with the wrong blocks.'" Priscilla continued. "Sometimes we can be fooled by false representations of reality and miss the real thing."

"I think I get it," said Mark. "Maybe when an atheist get so insistent on no-belief, he stubbornly refuses to budge from that position he has dug in with heels, and so can't see what is so obvious."

"Yes, that could be," said Beth, "But maybe an atheist has a point. I remember in one of my religious classes one of my teachers wrote this on the board: 'If a person tells me that he has a car which can do two hundred kilometres in one hour, I'll tell him to bring out the car and prove it. If you tell me that there is a God, I'll ask you to produce God to prove God's existence.' How would you respond to that challenge? The teacher got us in groups to discuss that and come up with solution."

Mark asked, "So, what did you decide, was there a proving or disproving? Did your group come up with an answer?"

"We came up with some, but I can't remember if any of us the right one," said Beth.

"Priscilla, what do you think?" asked Mark.

"I don't think anyone can claim to know God," said Priscilla, "nor would one want to know God in that way. One philosopher's view is you cannot know anything to perfection, especially a God. What I think a believer does not say is, 'I know God,' nor would he say, 'I see God' or 'I think there is a God.' But a believer can legitimately say instead, 'I believe in God.' God is a verb, not a noun."

"How so?" asked Mark.

Beth piped in, "Mark, you're always using that— 'how so?'"

"Well," Mark said impatiently, "I want to know how things work!"

Priscilla injected, "Right, Mark, by asking the how question, you can lead to what I'm going to say next, namely, we can know God only by what God does, moreover, when one only says, 'I believe in God,' I think what that person is saying, and rightly so, is this, 'I believe in God, because I believe God won't let me down.'"

"Kind of like my teammates on our football team—we believe in each other. No one is going to let the other down. We all have confidence in each other." Mark nodded in approval for what he just said.

Beth stared at Mark for some time. He began to look

unforgettable. Then turned to Priscilla. "There's got to be more to it than that! When I was in Sunday School—a long time ago—I memorized this: 'Now we know in part. But when perfection comes, partial knowledge will be abolished. Now we see dimly, as in a dark mirror. Then we will know completely as we are known now.' I'm not sure where that is in the Bible. But it is. Mark, you know that one."

"First Corinthians, somewhere," said Mark.

"You know that one?" Beth asked.

"I've heard of it," Mark muttered as he stared out across the lake.

"Well, maybe we can't say for sure we know all there is to know till . . ." Beth paused. "Till the end, even maybe then . . ."

Priscilla also stared across the lake, then all around her, then, looking down at Plato, said, "Belief in something, God perhaps, that's where we need to start, a leap of faith. Could it be when all is going well, we as creators forget about the Creator? In time, we forget God, and eventually may dismiss God as irrelevant or nonexistent. But when life takes different turns, as life inevitably does, then our tone often changes. Maybe we can't even decide we believe for sure, despite all that we've said, until our faith is tested. Maybe that's when we have a chance to see whether what we cling to stands the test.

"CS. Lewis put it this way: 'You never know how much you believe in anything until its truth or falsehood becomes a matter of life and death. It is easy to say you believe a rope to be strong and sound as long as you're merely using it to cord a box. But suppose you had to hang by that rope over a precipice. Wouldn't you then first discover how much you really trusted it? Only a real risk tests the reality of a belief." (C.S.Lewis 1952)

"But," Mark asked, "if you're talking about belief in that arena, then do we have to wait for a life and death moment to check to see if our belief is for real? Belief in what God does till proven otherwise would be less painful."

Priscilla said, "That's right, Mark, you got it. Atheism won't ease that kind of anxiety you're thinking of, any more than it can provide a refuge in the nasties of life or rob death of its sting. When we're young in years and feel invincible, death doesn't even enter our minds. It's then your observation rings even more true. For it's easy to flirt with atheism, dropping it only when we're in the presence of death. No wonder one writer noted, 'I buried my materialism in the grave of my father.'" Priscilla shifted gears a bit and said, "Let's suppose you don't have to wait to test the legitimacy of your belief in God. Maybe there is another way to talk about a belief in God that has to be about being PRACTICAL. Otherwise, *POOF . . .*"

"What?" Both Mark and Beth stared at Priscilla.

Priscilla said, "How's that for getting your attention! Worked with my students too. Anyway, GK Chesterton once said, "It is often supposed that when people stop believing in God, they believe in nothing. Alas, it's worse than that. When we stop believing in God, you believe anything. Ours is an age of vast unbelief, and yet an age which is pathetically willing to believe in anything given half a chance. " Priscilla continued. "In a play by Chekhov called *Three Sisters*, a person called Masha says, 'I think a human being has got to have some faith or at least he's to seek faith. Otherwise his life will be empty, empty. How can you live and not know why the cranes fly, why children are born, why the stars shine in the sky. You must either know why you live or nothingness matters. Everything's just wild grass." Chekhov 1901)

Having shared these great thinkers' ideas, Priscilla asked her two young friends what we thought of all that.

"Maybe it's practical to believe in God. Otherwise, we lose by default if we believe in nothing," said Mark

"That's right," said Beth, "and not to believe is running away from the big important questions that nature poses."

"I think you're both on the right track," Priscilla said, patting her dog's head.

"What do you think, Plato? They are very bright, right?" Turning then to the two with a smile, I went on to say, "I think that together, after our thought wondering and wandering, we're getting closer to where we want to be."

"Right," said Mark.

"Something like those geese circling there, looking for a place to land after having been foraging out in the grain fields. Something like that, right, Priscilla?" Beth said.

"Close. How about we read some thought in words I brought along. Gosh, sorry, for a moment, I thought I was back in the lecture hall. Anyway, maybe you'd be willing to indulge me by going along with the three of us, taking turns reading these passages; it takes us more than meeting together this week. Then after, if you wish, we can talk about whenever you happen to be passing through the park in the future. What do you think?"

Mark said, "Sure, that works for me."

"Great, let's do that," Beth added.

"Thanks, you two. Here they are then.

"One. 'After Einstein concluded a lecture on the Milky Way, a person asked him, 'If the world is so little and the universe is so great can we really believe that God pays any attention to us?' 'That,' replied the astronomer, 'depends entirely on how big a God you believe in.' Einstein surprised his fans when he was asked, 'Do you believe that absolutely everything can be expressed scientifically?' 'Yes,' he replied, 'it would be possible, but it would make no sense. It would be descriptive without meaning, as if you described Beethoven's symphony as variations of wave pressure.' (Einstein n.d.)

Two. Some people of different faith stances may say when one finally sees the futility of pursuing material wealth or creature comforts, or satiating of one's appetites, that person looks elsewhere and discovers God was there all the time, ignored but very real" Priscilla continued to share with the youngsters the readings.

Three. "A person who gave up agnosticism and found his way into a place of worship said, 'I wanted to know the answer of good and evil, what was unbearable was to think that there is no moral awakening, that we creep from moment to moment deceiving ourselves, sometimes guilty and remorseful, sometimes happy, but never knowing the answer, never seeing things as a whole." (Thoreau 2008)

"Four. 'Seeing the immense design of the world, I explained one image of wonder mirrored by another image of wonder, the pattern of fern and feather echoed by the frost on the windowpane, the six rays of the snowflake mirrored by the rock crystals six rayed eternity. Then I asked herself, were those shaped, moulded by blindness? Who then shall teach me doubt?'

"Five. 'What can be more foolish than to think that all this rare fabric of heaven and earth could come by chance, when all the skill of art is not able to make an oyster? To see rare effects, and no cause, a motion. Without a mover, a circle without a centre, a time without an eternity, a second, without a first.

"Six. The experience of life nearly always works toward the confirmation of faith. It is the total significance of life that reveals God to humans, and life only can do his. Neither thought, nor demonstration, nor miracle, but only life weaving us threads of daily toil and trial and joy into a pattern will at last inscribe the name of God (Sitwell n.d.)

"Seven. 'Don't close all the doors to on faith yet. Live a little more, experience much, and you will eventually discover a God who has been walking with you all the time. You just may not have known it, for if neither intellect and logic nor the wonder of creation will convince you, there is a living God experience that will go on.

The following week after we had read through the passages, Beth and Mark entered the park in great expectation of meeting our mentor. They were very excited and had so much that they wanted to share. *Hamlet's* "to be or not to be" had taken on so much more meaning! They looked down the path, searching for the familiar figure of Priscilla sitting with Plato. But . . . they weren't there. The park bench was empty.

A Spirit Lake Park bench plaque read:

In Memory of Priscilla and Plato.
1 Corinthians 13:11-13

It Happened

At a police station, an old lady sat, blank faced; no one seemed to know she was there. Then out she went, feeling she needed to find someone, didn't know who or why. "Big building, I'll go there. Someone came out, I slipped in, an elevator, vague about that, *ring*, door slid open, strange but familiar. I crammed in with others, *ring*, door opened, I pushed by out into a hall, stairs, searching, climbing, elevator, down, door opened, outside. Question: "You live here?" Let back in, climbed more stairs, then on one floor, long hall I faintly remembered shuffling up and down, somewhere safe, yes, that was why I kept going. A door opened, a man stepped out, a place he lived in, I thought. He was way down the hall but now walking toward me, a face of recognition, a big smile, open arms wide, not knowing why but his hugs felt good, safe

I said, "I want to go home now."

"Okay, let's."

Got there, he pushed the buzzer, an intercom voice, yes, I felt good again, first time in a long time, Then hugs, home, I knew way, the elevator stopped at the second floor, I didn't know why, but this was it. Without a word of gibberish, I felt safe, and knowing, up and down the hall I went, in and out of rooms off the hall, staring blank faced, more hugs and kisses. I walked, sat, slept, oh so tired. Nights and days, more of the same, then I said, "Well, that enough of that, it's time."

I slept, pain, then no pain, eyes opened, closed, soft music, whispers. I knew love all around me, breathe in and out, pause, stop, started again, darkness, crying, opened eyes, saw tears. I reached out a hand held another, closed eyes, darkness, nothing. Then a warm glow, vague figures blending with mist, twin brother felt near, knew I was safe, okay in the formless presence of others at peace.

Chapter 6: It Can Go Either Way

Sometimes people in the Park got hooked into conversation where the big questions of life were explored. The park gives people the opportunity to stop and reflect on what life is really all about, leading to gaining meaningful insights, especially after the death of a loved one.

Some might say the chief reason for doing things is to relieve boredom and that's all there really is. Others might say, "No, it's to satisfy one's appetites, or to be entertained.

One book in the Bible, Ecclesiastes (3: 1-15) presents a ho hum attitude about life, suggesting life is really a futile chore where one is obliged to get through as best one can, given there are many experiences one can't avoid. That blissful, fatalistic way may cause a disconnect with nature and its potential to deliver surprises, both good and bad.

An incident happened in an Arctic community where a young father and son left their home to walk parallel to the shore on a freezing winter day. (The father either missed hearing the weather report of an impending storm, or ignored it.)

When we started out, the sun was shining, and visibility was good. A raging storm developed, with a strong wind blowing toward the shore, pushing the father and son from their sides. The father apparently used that wind as a guide.

Unfortunately, the wind changed to the opposite direction without the father realizing it. Consequently, he, with his son, instead of hugging the shoreline as he thought he was doing, walked further away from safety onto the vast sea ice. Their bodies, when found, were huddled together. The father's parka wrapped around his son.

The Crazy Fisherman

In a book titled *Once Upon a Little Town* by MacDonald Coleman, there is a chapter called, "The Crazy Fisherman." In it, the reader hears a youngster talking to Mr. Orchard. Everyone knew that Ben Orchard was slightly 'crazy, loony in the old beano.' But after reading the chapter, one wonders, was he really? For in the conversation, Ben Orchard poses the profound perennial question that haunts us all: "What are we living for?"

The conversation goes on; old Ben suggests an answer.

The story ends with an interesting surprise. The young-ster watches old Ben fishing where even he, a youngster, knows there are no fish. He hears Ben say finally, when challenged with that fact, "Look, kid, I'll show you some-thing. Look at my fishing rod, for a fish-less creek you should always use a fish-less fishing rod."

Then the kid says, "But you'll never catch a fish!"

"Yes I will. Anyway, I'm a vegetarian and I don't eat fish. But yes, I catch fish here. I caught you this afternoon, and you've been a very pleasant, nice fish. Come and see me any time you like." (Coleman 1979)

Chapter 7: Bus Riders' Stories

I found revisiting these stories helpful to reconnect with others outside my grieving, just as the Spirit Lake Park stories helped me reconnect with nature. I found both together very therapeutic.

Aging Pet Lover

"Turtles."

"Yes, pet turtles."

"Where?"

"In the garden in the summer, house in winter."

"How big? Big as dinner plates?"

"No. Bigger! We're as old as me," I said.

I listened in on the back and forth sharing by two strangers to each other sitting side by side on the bus.

"Have you other pets?"

"Dogs, two of us, big! Live in the backyard."

"Must be cold in the winter."

"No, insulated dog house, "

"For both?"

"Yes, but the one's trouble. Still, we make do."

"What does your husband think about all that?"

"Oh, he's okay. Has enough to think about, stopped smoking when his dad died." I went on to say, "He's a pet."

"His dad was?"

"No, my husband is. Had a heart attack, not the man he was. But he gets along okay in the house."

"You're there with him a lot since the attack?"

"No. I work at a bookstore/coffee shop. Serve coffee and stuff. Used to own a bookstore, but the big boys pushed me out. Couldn't compete with the big chains. Loved books, but really the ones I love dearly are at home."

"The books?"

"No, my pets," she said. "And what about you?"

Contented Old Trucker

The wrinkles on his weathered face and his squinting watery eyes added to his grimacing, painful appearance. He did get his contorted body up the bus stairs, pausing to get his breath before he began his arthritic journey down the aisle. Now and then he'd grab the armrest of a seat for balance before searching, searching for an empty seat in the packed bus. Seeing one beside me, he paused, and with a determined look and extreme concentration, lurched towards it. I stood; he almost knocked me over in trying to shift his big body between seats. He clung to a bundle, barely getting his short arms around it. Finally, his efforts paid off. He sank down into the window seat, his bundle in his lap.

Despite the cold, he wiped perspiration off his brow. The sweat had run along the side of his blue-veined nose. He looked all in. "Thought I'd not make it," he said. "Those pins don't have what it takes to carry me around anymore, not like when I trucked and lugged heavy milk cans." Then began a long story of how he trucked a few years. "One day a friend who worked at a dairy said he'd put out a good word for him there, so he could make better money with less to do. He got the job, and said, "My old lady was happy. Now we got a garden, a house I fixed up, and it's all paid for, some grandkids, and some time to fish. I'm retired, you know."

We were coming into Vulcan when his story trailed off. When most people bushed by to step off for a break in the gas station store, he nudged me to let him out of his cramped space. I stayed put and drifted off, only to be nudged again. This time he juggled in shaky hands a big drink and napkin-wrapped bun around sausage splattered with mustard, ketchup, and onions—the works!

To my dismay his smacking was accompanied by a few belches, My grimacing face didn't deter him from beginning where he left off, giving me a blow-by-blow detailed description of all the work he had done, and how his bosses found his work good.

And so he rambled on while I, with my head down, intensified my intrigue with the technical attributes of the bag in which I had spewed up my supper.

Finally, we arrived, He thanked me for the nice visit.

Respected Elder

Two people stepped onboard, looking left and right, heads down; speaking Chinese, They sought out seats. He shouted. She spoke quietly in a reassuring voice. He was very old and feeble.

Seeing this very touching drama unfold, I recalled watching parents make sure children, if travelling alone, were settled and safe. Once young, now old, once treated as a strong man, now as a child, the Chinese gentleman received the parent love from one who once was his child.

When his daughter left the bus, he shifted about, seeking a comfortable position. With his head against the seat back and his hand groping to press the button to push it back, he stiffened and strained with no success. He turned, leaned over the arm rest, twisted his neck this way and that, peered, looking puzzled, for the reluctant button, playing hide-and-seek.

Across the aisle, a younger man looked his way, and, without a word, waved his hands to indicate how to succeed. Finally, he went over, smiled at the old man, pushed and yanked, and the seat went back. The old man nodded a thank you. And rested.

One Having Courage to Be

His face was weathered and deeply lined, and his big hands blue-veined with fingers gnarled and swollen. His story? One who gave his all and left it all behind, not on a playing field or rink, but in a cruel mine. Now his best years were behind him, and his memories, like the lines etched into his face, could have left him bitter and sad.

Well, his making conversation showed it hadn't. He had a forty-year-old mentally-challenged son living at home with him. "But he does alright," he said. "Makes thousands of bits of things for a local manufacturer each month. My son also goes with me fishing, and ski-ing. We have two dogs. My son loves us. So do I. They go everywhere with us."

I never asked about his wife, but I did about where he was going.

"To see my granddaughter skate. She goes all over, and I try to get to as many of her events as I can, don't mind the bus." He smiled with a look of pride. Life's good. My son too."

Farmer's Wife

She looked worn but wiry, with a sparkle in her eyes and

a weathered, friendly face that wore a smile well. Our talk began about the weather, but like a Chinook blowing in, picked up, talking about crops, water, farm, machinery, and fertilizers. She said, "I knew about all that. Though that wasn't the way it was at first. I had started out as a city girl. That changed when a young farmer stepped into the office where I worked. He kept coming back till I left there for good, ending up a farmer's wife.

"You learn how to drive tractor and truck?" I asked.

"No. My place was in the house and in the garden. Besides, my husband had four brothers. One lived with us; the others had different farms nearby. We worked together for years. I wasn't needed in their doings."

"And after?"

"The brothers got out of farming. Our kids didn't want anything to do with the farm. So, we moved into town. Travelled a bit. Then my husband got sick, died on me. I moved into a condominium."

"Like it?" I asked.

"Lots! Us girls, my friends, we walk and play bridge, never a dull moment!"

"You're going to Calgary?"

"Yes, to visit some of my grandkids, babysit them often. My kids don't come out here much. We have our own lives. I go to them. They're busy. That's okay. I don't mind the bus. Don't drive except around town."

One Too Old to Work, Too Young to Retire

She sat in the seat above the open door, beside the driver. So debonair, dressed expensively, She appeared out of place in a bus full mostly of young people struggling to make ends meet, either at college or sweating it out in Banff's serving industry. Who was this woman sitting like a real lady, her firm, ample body accentuating the finery of her garments?

After a comment about the road conditions, we began the "Where are you from," and "What do you do ?"

"I worked in public relations for years. Husband died after we moved out to the country. We built a big house. It had everything. "It looked like I had as well. Before he died, we golfed, hobnobbed with the local elite. Lots of parties."

"And now?"

"I'm thinking of moving back to Calgary," she says. "But to do what? I'm too old to go back to work. And now, since he died, I'm too young to bury myself in the country. Money is no problem. It's time. What do I do with the time?"

At the next stop, I leaned back as more young people scurried onboard with purposeful looks on their faces. Did she have that same purposeful look on her face years ago? "Yes, when young. Now?

Tree Faller's Wife

The knitting bag lay open on the seat, another below on the

floor. Searching for an aisle seat and spotting the empty one next to the knitting bag, she sat. Someone had claimed the window seat. That was evident. But someone would also be back before the bus set out after a break stop.

When the bag's owner took her seat and settled, I spoke. "Looks like you've been on the road a long time."

"Since seven this morning."

I say, "Sounds like you've come a long way. To see your kids?"

"Nope."

That didn't get me anywhere, I thought.

I tried again. "Calgary's a nice place. Be there in about an hour and a half."

"I hate it," she muttered.

"What?"

"Calgary."

Here we go again, I thought, "You hate it because . . . ?"

"Grew up and moved to a nice little town."

"How was that for you?"

"Great!" I smiled. "Had a school caretaker job for years. Loved the kids."

"You found folks in your job become real friends to the kids, and tried you as one to share troubles with?"

"That's true," she said.

"You left though."

"Daughter in Calgary, so I thought I'd try something new there."

"Going there now to live?"

"For a while, just coming back from visiting mother. Lives alone in the country."

Dad died."

"Nice place to live?"

"Grew up there, wildlife all over the place, otherwise quiet," she said, looking wistful.

"Like a sanctuary."

"Was till fires close by, only road in clogged with vehicles. Some fighting fires, others just gawking. Curious as hell. Problem, Father needed the road clear for an ambulance. He was a mess, health-wise. Heart, the works. We were in danger of losing him then, hordes of people. The fire was close to our house."

"Was he okay?"

"Oh yeah, He didn't die because we couldn't clear the road to get him to the hospital. It was after, he just gave up, and that was that."

"Your dad farmed?"

"No, he was a tree faller, later had his own small mill."

"Logging can be tough?"

"Yes, but Dad was tough, even though he had only one leg, lots of mended broken bones, back pain. Still he refused to quit till near the end. Smoker, too. Times in hospital with it. Couldn't tell him anything. Just like my husband."

"He's a logger too?"

"Was a faller, now has a small mill on the Island. We're separated but still keep in touch. Everything's in my name. He's also in bad shape. But keeps going. Tough there too, lumber, fishing, lots out of work. But he also had his hobby, burls, builds furniture. Had an attic in his shop, full of burls drying out to work on. The house was full of wood he'd milled: did some fancy wood stuff. It's everywhere in the house, cabinets, floors, bedstead. I got so tired of wood here, there, everywhere. Damn wood!"

"Now?"

"Sold the place when we separated. Still see each other's friends; I now can't tell him anything. He drinks, smokes, even though, like Dad, he's in and out of hospital. Half a lung gone. He gets back out, first thing, got a cig hanging out of his mouth. I gave up."

"You miss it out where he lives?"

"Some. My daughter goes back to the mountains to get a fix when I can't take Calgary. But I'm better out here. It's the climate, drier. I've got arthritis, am a diabetic too, That's why you hear the rattle of my munchies. Gals at work—I work in a department store—They watch out for me when I get confused and show the signs, They say to me, 'You go and eat now.' Got to be careful. So I go to the lunch room and just about choke on smoke. What can I do! I stay because the pay's good. Well. Not good as my old caretaker's job, but still, it's okay. Had an offer to go work at a private school to do my old kind of work. Said no, don't like driving in Calgary. So, I don't. Thinking of selling my car. Daughter drives me to work and picks me up after. I'll be alright. Daughter and me buying a house together. Just us and two dogs. When I quit work, I'll get my sewing machine out and do more sewing."

"Using what you got there?"

"Yes, this one bag is full of material. Going to make dresses for the two grandkids."

"You look uncomfortable with that bag on your lap. Do you want me to put it up in the luggage rack?"

"No, we're getting close to home. You do this trip lots?"

"Yes."

"For business?"

"Yes."

Old Cowboy Landlord

A deep-throated, gargling sound gave me a bit of a start. I had just sagged down to lean on the seat back. The sound could have come from a tobacco spitting cowboy talking to his horse. I was partially right. Turning around and looking over the seat back, I saw a sagging, grey, watery-eyed fellow. He did wear a cowboy hat, jeans, and mother-of-pearl, dome-buttoned shirt.

But then his question: "Where yam from?"

I answered, "From the city."

Scratching, shifting his paunch over his belt, he blurted, "Well, I'm from the country, and I got a cowboy hat, but I'm not a cowboy. I'm a rancher and work with my dad."

Looking at this weathered old fellow, I thought, *Goodness, if he's still at it, I'd like to meet the tough old bird whom he calls Dad. And who took him out of school when just a kid.*

He wanted to talk. So I listened.

He'd just come back across the USA border, having been down checking up on the state of the house he owns down there. His renters took off, wrecked the place, and he had to make it right.

"It's tough doing business at a distance. And that's it." His voice trailed off, and I turned my head to stare over the seat in front of me. I heard, "Nice knowing you."

I closed my eyes and listened to the rain doing a line dance on the top of the bus. It sounded like the pastures were getting a good soaking.

Absentee Dad

One Sunday evening, I began a conversation with a lean, rugged young man. He didn't hesitate to share his journey. "Been down on the rigs, got a woman down there, and two kids. Trying to get them into Canada. They.re Mexican. I love my old lady, but it's not much fun, she down there, and me up here most of the time.

Now been making big bucks."

The guy went on, looking at me with a thin, drawn face

and sadness in his eyes. He showed me pictures of his wife and kids. They e looked poor and pathetic, as did he, and despite the money that he said he'd earned, he said, "It's tough to keep it, with all the bills to pay for my truck and booze. A guy has to have some fun, don't he?"

I said, "I don't think I know."

"Hell," he said, "I don't think I know myself either."

Feeling I didn't want to go there with him, I slapped on my headphones and sought sleep.

He stared at the window, a mirror darkened by the night.

Distant One

"May I sit here?" She pointed to the window seat. slim and appeared fit. Her blonde hair, high cheekbones, and grey eyes gave her a sports magazine model look.

I was curious about how she would occupy her time h on the trip from Lethbridge to Calgary. Would she read? Would she don headphones and isolate herself, listening to music? Would I try to concentrate? Stare out the window?

What? To my surprise, she spent the whole trip staring straight ahead, looking neither left nor right. It was as if she were a department store mannequin, revealing only her profile. Strange! What goes on in a person's mind when in an in-between state of mind?

Private Couple with Child

The two with proud stoic looks, well-dressed, moved gracefully down the bus aisle. The mother carried her child, the man the luggage and baby bag. They sank in the seats across from me.

The dad took the child, stood him between his legs, and held the child's arms up to support him. The little one lunged forward, giggling. Mom and Dad didn't smile. Neither of their brown and tired faces showed any feelings as their r child's chubby feet made a few little steps.

Sitting across from the couple, I looked from the child to the parents, and back to the child. The two stared ahead.

Impressed with their baby's efforts, I said, "He's doing very well."

The couple's faces neither smiled nor frowned. It was as if their baby's actions were private between the three of them, and I intruded..

I wondered, was that much the same when non-natives attempt to bridge the gap between themselves and indigenous people? It appeared that despite all the water that had gone under the bridge, at least this couple kept their pride of self and race. I could share space on a bus, but would I ever be able to come at least halfway across the gap?

Two Kids that Clicked

A comfort level seemed apparent on one trip. Two young-sters stepped onto the bus. Both were familiar and comfortable with the bus. Neither spoke at first, though one sat right behind the other. The one, awkward and stringy, appeared all legs and arms in perpetual motion, where the other, a little peaked ten-year-old, sat quietly, deeply engrossed in a pocket computer game, totally ignoring all around him.

The restless one played with a similar game, but curious, he snaked his body, stretching it around the aisle seat to look over the quieter boy's shoulder. "That yours?"

"No, it's my dad's."

"Want to play with my game, and I'll play with yours?"

With neither a word nor a smile, the quiet boy turned around, exchanged games, and slumped down again in his seat, his little nail-bitten fingers dancing around on the game board. The restless one octopuses his way back into his seat, and he, too, kept his busy hands and mind affixed to the fascination of the board.

I saw two boys, one quiet and introverted, the other restless and precocious, sharing, neither asking each other why or how come. This showed me a truth. Here is the now, that's all there is. The self, another person, and a shared space, and that can be enough. Sometimes no questions, no explanations, are needed.

Hockey Player's Mom

I sat beside a woman who turned out to be the mother of, would you believe it, Tony Twist! Who is Tony Twist? "Why, a Canadian expert to USA hockey, former member of St Louis Blues.

"He was, till a motorcycle accident destroyed his hockey career. He wasn't the best skater," she said, "but he knew what he wanted, and he went out and got it. Now he owns some restaurants down there.

"Heading to Calgary, passing through Banff from home. I'm going to babysit one ferret and two dogs for my daughter."

Chapter 8: High Arctic Intensity

The High Arctic was a remembered experience, a source of wonderment, intensity, and surprise, one where reconnecting with nature and others happened, and in remembering, it enhanced my will to live on. The clarity and intensity of the Arctic's nature and inhabitants could not be matched.

This account of Lesley's and my brief High Arctic experience is one of many moves and stays that may have contributed to her depression, dementia, and eventual demise, but also, it was inherently good, for the gift of hospitality and inherent kindness of the Grise Fiord Inuit residents, and of two lifelong friends, Tom and Midge, who offered support where nature and friendship meets intensity.

How It Began and Unfolded as an Unforgettable Life Experience

I and I spent three great years at Norway House, Manitoba. But eventually, we decided to make a move. The federal government was looking for people to teach among the Inuit; I applied for a transfer. Having received an invitation to attend an interview in Winnipeg, I jumped at the chance to see what it was all about. Lesley and I looked over the package of information before I left for an interview' Lesley said she would go "anywhere but there," pointing to a settlement on the southern tip of Ellesmere Island.

I said, "Right!" and I was off to meet Gordon Dewitt, the school superintendent and another official. They invited me and others to our hotel suite.

Mr. Devitt gave a little talk about teaching up north. Then he told us it was good to take some plastic artificial flowers with us. After, he took me aside and asked if I'd teach—you guessed it—at Grise Fiord on Ellesmere Island. Thinking I wouldn't get an offer to go anywhere else, I said yes. Arriving back at Norway House, I broke the news to Lesley. She reluctantly agreed to go with me. Thus began our move even further north, stopping at Resolute Bay before flying into Grise.

The Beaver aircraft stood on the tarmac at Resolute. It looked so very small, too small to pack in our toddler sons Andrew and Mark, Olaf, the new engineer, myself, and our worldly possessions. Just the thought of us all crammed into that tiny craft, hanging in the air on the way to Grise Fiord, over Arctic open water, made me shudder. What if that single engine conked out? What then? Dare we go and risk our children's lives?

We saw Resolute disappear. We were off, sharing space with a few mail bags and cartons. The pilot, unlike many I had flown with, after take-off didn't pull out a book to read, or ignore his fearful passengers. He graciously passed around candy, smiled most reassuringly behind his cookie-cutter moustache and sleepy eyes. Now and then he pointed where we might look through the Plexiglas at icebergs, stony beaches, and white whales.

Eventually, we saw over the plane's engine cowling, a few dots in the distance in a bead-like pattern along the tip of a fjord. There it was, Grise Fiord, about nine hundred or so miles from the north pole. Our pilot circled the small settlement, nosed the plane down to land, then revved his engine and swung around behind a rocky obstruction, obliterating sight of downtown Grise. Where was he going to land, no airstrip, no clear smooth open place in sight? The answer? Right there, on the rocky beach formed by low tide. Not there!? Oh, yes! The little Beaver mushed in, stalled at the point of landing, bumped and leaped up into the air before settling down to wait. Soon, around the bend came a freighter canoe with two tiny little people that reminded me of two of the seven dwarfs. They piled us and the plane's cargo into their canoe. The pilot gunned the Beaver's engine and was away, leaving us alone in a very strange place of intense blues and ice. The canoe ricocheted off bobbing pieces of ice, and despite hearing the canoe boards crack and groan, our driver wheeled around the corner, laughing all the way. Scary, to say the least!

Like the Beaver aircraft and the little men who picked us up, the settlement also looked so small. What did we see? One RCMP house, a tiny duplex for two special constables and their large families, and one garage-like co-op store. Along the shore a school complex with three wings, a teacherage, classroom, and engineer's quarters. A power house, and about a dozen very small structures housing, the Inuit families, designed from a chicken coop plan, completed the picture. The theory was that since the "Eskimos" lived in tents and igloos of diminutive size, it would feel right to house Inuit in such creations. Some Inuit families who received the material for those on the annual sealift evidently saw the possibility of straight walls rather than the indented ones shown on the plans. Thus , practical as they were, made more interior space than the southern Kadlunat (non-Inuit) engineers thought would be "just right."

The teacherage, when built, could also have used a little Inuit northern know-how. For scary were the winds that crashed down the fjord, forcing our living room picture window to bulge inward. The builders oriented the teacherage to stare right into the path of the wind rushing down the fjord. We would pull the window drapes and hope that the glass, bowing in and out, wouldn't harm our two toddlers, Andrew and Mark.

The school complex stood on stilts on a gravel pad. Had it not, the permafrost would have melted from the heat of the building, and we'd be sunk. Standing on stilts had one drawback, though. The whole business could lift and fly away across the sea ice, the way a few of our bed sheets did. Those, frozen like boards, cartwheeled into the distance after Lesley hung s on the clothesline to dry.

Living in the residence did offer unique experiences. With no room in the kitchen, the surviving bed sheets brought in from outdoors stood stiff and proud in the living room. Eventually thawed out and flopped over to join other bedcovers that frequently stuck to the bedroom's metal walls festooned with frost-coated rivet-like knobs.

The water used to wash our boys' cloth diapers, for bathing, washing dishes, and cleaning floors all came from an ice melting tank. Olaf and Sam Willy fetched the ice on a sled from icebergs in the winter. The melting tank's electric coil couldn't melt the ice fast enough. For Olaf, who kept the power generators operating, among other things, loved to keep his body immaculately clean with long showers. He habitually questioned Lesley's use of so much water. I would repeat our household's litany of needs. He would say "Yah, yah," puff his cigar vigorously, and make a hasty retreat, only to repeat the ritual again in subsequent days.

Olaf did have the help of Sam Willy and even a big "husky," as some Inuit men were called back then. That boy with a deep, loud voice, proud of his strength, would tackle the primary reader with sincerity and good humour. Yet at least once I had to stimulate his interest in school. Going to his home to fetch him out of bed, only to find him dressed and curled up, clinging tightly to his alarm clock. That was it. He welcomed with open arms my suggestion that he would learn more helping Sam Willy and Olaf fill the ice melting tank.

Our whole school complex heating system depended on electricity. If it shut down, all would freeze up within an hour or so, leaving us in deep trouble! It differed from the RCMP quarters that operated on simpler principles.

I thought that I kept my worrying over our precarious position to myself, I and the kids need not engage in the nasty game of thinking, *What if this went wrong, or that?* Mark had run high temperatures with tonsillitis. Deep down, Lesley and I feared not only for our children's lives, but also for the lives of the other people's children. With no doctor or nursing station for hundreds of miles, could a plane come cutting through the heavy mist and fog that often remained trapped in the fjord? It really ticked

Lesley off that the RCMP wouldn't think of sending a wife or kids so far north, yet, our department (DIANA) had no qualms about doing so. Still, I tried to keep Lesley's spirits up, helped by the caring Inuit and reassuring presence of the two Mounties, Tom and Lorne. Lorne, six-five and over two hundred pounds, often sat at the kitchen table comparing cookie recipes with Lesley while I taught next door. His cookies were big like him, saucer size. Tom's experiences seemed more exciting. Once while Tom was on patrol, his dogs took off on him, arriving home before he did. He had stopped to untangle the dog team lines, normally fanned out in front of his Komatik. Into the teacherage he came, face and moustache all glistening with frost. With a twinkle in his eyes, unmoved by the mishap, he chuckled about an episode in Dickens's Pickwick Papers that he'd been reading.

Lesley and I got some comfort from Tom and Lorne's frequent visits; They offered support and encouragement.

Sundays, while Tom holed up with a good book or a visit with Olaf, Lorne, Lesley and I would tackle a bit of scripture. Lorne had a thing about enjoying descriptions of the architecture of heaven. I and Lesley felt we had better things in the Bible to ponder over. Lorne had a different way of interpreting the Bible than we did. But still, that was okay.

Once Tom and Lorne had a serious concern. What would cause these two capable men with all the resources of the RCMP at their fingertips, share with Lesley and me that concern? They were deeply troubled. dealing with a seriously ill baby, having only immediately available Merk's *Manual*, the medical dispenser's northern Bible.

"Don't Worry Be Happy" was a song I heard, containing a good attitude for surviving mentally in the Arctic. Good food helped the morale. We were satisfied with our food supply for the most part. Huge containers, four times the size of square hay bales, arrived via the sealift. They contained rations, canned and dried foods, that, if eaten according to the dietician that requisitioned the stuff, provided sufficient nutrition for our bodies. onion flakes, big square cans of stringy roast beef and pork—the strands of which you could weave into rope— assorted canned goods, tea, sugar, flour, powdered eggs, the basics, and other assorted canned meats, and three very scrumptious items: Danish bacon, Danish butter, and Baker's chocolate.

All great for the body The mind? That was something else.

Lesley and I and our children were sometimes guests at Tom and Lorne's table, an added morale booster during dark times.

While at Grise Fiord, the new maple leaf Canadian flag was hoisted high for the first time on the RCMP and school flag poles. That met with wide smiles, but also confused looks, from many who had been accustomed to the Union Jack. After all, were not we, the people of Grise way up north, to show the flag and assert Canadian sovereignty over that part of the Arctic? That question at the time didn't occur to me as a hot issue. Peering out the snowflake-frosted window of the school at the flag often did cause me to feel homesick for the south. The flag evoked memories of warmer more hospitable places, where that hoisted new emblem caused fewer puzzled faces and more cheers. I always felt the new flag looked a lot like the Maple Leaf lard label, only red instead of blue. Lesley, very proud of being a Canadian, often chastised me about the cynical views I shared with tongue in cheek.

Lesley and I often shared private thoughts. We had been curious about the Inuit people from northern Quebec. They apparently had come by sealift a few years before we arrived. Now they lived in Grise with three brothers with families from Pond Inlet, whom we understood were to teach them how to survive and hunt in the High Arctic. One older Quebec Inuit woman shared how she and others felt when first arrived in such a dark, foreign, inhospitable place. "We thought we had sent us here to die," she said.

Nevertheless, despite that harsh beginning, the resilience of the human spirit revealed itself. The Quebec men and women no doubt compared notes with the Pond Inlet people on how they differed in what they did to survive. The fan hitch for hitching dogs to the komatiks seemed best. If a dog needed to crap or pee, he didn't hold the whole gang up. If a dog fell through the ice, the others may drag him out or the driver could cut the one loose to save the rest. One wondered why the Quebec women insisted on continuing to use the HBC plaid shawls instead of adopting the amautik parka to keep themselves and babies warm. Was it Arctic custom or cultural pride? Survival was of first importance. Out of necessity, one man, who suffered from ulcers, needed his adolescent son with him when out hunting. Another often took his son out of school to either pass on the art of survival and killing for food, or to develop a father and son bond, or both.

I heard a story of one such fellow and his young son, Looty, who got separated, and found themselves in a predicament. A polar bear ended up between father and son. Looty or the father shot the bear. I believe our family got that bear skin, or one like it. After it was tanned and mounted, Andrew and Mark found great joy sliding down its head. They—as the only children of Cree ancestry possibly ever to step out into the High Arctic—would never have the experience of shooting a polar bear. The closest we got to being like the Inuit was wearing the crochet, tasselled toques, and parkas with the pointed hoods. The tips of the hoods, it's been said, were for God to be able to pull his people up to heaven.

Andrew and Mark, if Inuit, would have had adapted

names represented as Endorsee, and Marko see. The school register list included Moshe, Peepeelee, and more with "ee" endings. I had heard that the RCMP who registered births once imposed a rule that long names containing a repetition of vowels would be translated into English spelling. There seemed little difference between how this and how and customs officers greeted immigrants to Canada, solved the problem of pronunciation and writing out names. Both took liberties. However, I also heard that parents themselves sometimes caused their children to carry names based on performance in the infant or toddler stage. For instance, one runny-nosed little guy's name, when translated into English, meant "guts," possibly short for "greedy guts," to describe his enthusiastic eating habits.

Tom, Lorne and our two RCMP specials, who were the "policee," went on patrols with the specials assigned by the powers that be, and by Inuit custom, to look after whoever ventured forth into the High Arctic. I have a hunch the Inuit viewed us whites as little children to be watched over. It has been said they ostracize those who didn't look after characters from the south.

Tom and Lorne respected our keepers. Yet Tom also could enjoy the humour presented by Peameenee, one "special" who most of the time cut quite a figure. Those "specials" and families showed an unusual ability to get along so well together. Although practically lived in each other's laps all winter, still packed up a huge komatiks and canoes and headed out to holiday together on spring hunting and fishing excursions. I wondered how the Inuit could live close together without suffering cabin fever. Perhaps the reason was and is that they always displayed very highly sophisticated manners and customs. They seem to share a great respect for each other's personal space and feelings and avoid conflict at all costs.

I did wonder how the Quebeckers and the Pond Inlet people dealt with their two different dialects. Despite the differences, Tom, for one, did his best to handle both. Nevertheless, he did intimate there was only so much ice, snow, fishing, and hunting talk that one could do to sustain a conversation about snowed-in igloos while on patrols. Inevitably, starving for other topics to bandy about, he got around to Lesley and me quite often. We appreciated Tom and Lorne's company during the long months of darkness. We'd open the drapes in the morning to darkness, sometimes an intense dark, deep blue, a haunting huge moon, and no sun. Then summer and no night, none at all! It was then that many went around, bug-eyed, on a natural, perpetual high. At all hours of the night people would be busy and about. I often heard children giggling and twittering at three or four o'clock in the morning, having a good time on the swings. "Oh, if they would only go to sleep," I'd mumble to myself. They did when in class. Heads on their desks, they slumbered, slowly forcing their blackberry eyes open when

I interrupted their dreams. The solution was to get outdoors. We did. Desks found themselves planted firmly on the gravel outside. I thought up a geography lesson that involved running from place to place. I identified a big piece of the schoolyard, saying to the kids, "This is Baffin and Ellesmere Island. Here is Grise Fiord. There is Pond Inlet, and there is Arctic Bay, Broughton Island, Pangnirtung, Frobisher Bay, Cape Dorset, Igloolik, and so on." I placed a flag representing each settlement in geographical proximity to each other to model the way they would be situated spatially on Baffin Island. Then the big moment came, "Alright, now when I call out a settlement's name, you race to it." It was a less strenuous task for me to call the names than it was for the children to run to the flags. Soon they were puffing and laughing about the whole novel way of learning about their part of Canada. I felt good about finding the Inuit view of play, not who got there first or who won a race. That didn't matter much. Just the joy of doing it together was enough.

I had concluded some time ago that people have different learning styles. Inuit children, because of their active, outdoor lives, would learn more effectively through body movement in space, visually, and through touch. Besides, learning should be fun. I, for one, didn't do well in school back when the lecture method was prominent. It was not until I reached university, where I was free to learn using my own style, that I succeeded.

I clearly got the impression, in the short time that I

lived among the people, that for their children, learning how to survive was of first and foremost importance. I saw toddlers playing with axes and other sharp instruments. The parents, rather than taking away potential harm saying, "Don't do that, you'll hurt yourself," would give children of all ages the opportunity to hurt, to fail, and learn from that. I saw children playing by tide cracks; if slipped and fell into us, we'd be goners. When I asked the parents why they let their children risk their lives that way, told me that if a child or teen didn't have enough sense and skill to survive, it was better to find out sooner than later, rather than risk the lives of others as a grown up, for members of the community relied on each other for survival.

With our constant concern for our Andrew and Mark, it was hard for Lesley and me to accept that many of the youngsters wouldn't even arrive in adulthood strong and vigorous enough to survive in the High Arctic. Yes, they had seal and caribou, but was that enough to ensure a balanced diet? I recall identical twins. One had gone south to a hospital at a very early age, the other remained with her parents at Grise. The day came, after many years down south, when the girl, now healthy, returned to her parents in Grise. What a difference there was between the two. The child from the south, with cheeks aglow, seemed bigger, and very animated. The twin who had remained in Grise, in comparison, looked smaller and less lively.

The parents did the best they could in the High Arctic to provide. Yet the difference was evident. I couldn't help but wonder what the factors were that made the difference.

I did know that the mortality rate in the Arctic among the people was so great that Lorne or Tom somehow appointed me as acting coroner. It was not a joke. Nevertheless, with obviously no training in that job, I merely had the role of viewing a body and confirming with the RCMP that person was dead. One child, I recall, died of meningitis. That I could believe, because of the way the infant's body was contorted. In seeing that child,

The visitation of death came even closer to home when Sam Willy told me he was taking some time off to go up into the mountain. It was not really a mountain but, resembling the Rock of Gibraltar, just might well have been, for it towered over the settlement.

"Why, Sam Willy?"

"My baby died, and I will bury her."

"I'm so sorry!"

"Amiah," he said, meaning, "It can't be helped."

Fatalism may have been the only way that those fine people could survive in the harsh climate, so far away from medical help. The old cliché that death lurks everywhere was so true. One day I climbed that "mountain" and stood on its peak. For fun I formed stones into K+L, thinking some tourists would someday climb to that spot, and at first believe he or I stood where no southerner has stood before, only to be very surprised.

Just as I finished, and was walking backwards to admire my work, something told me to turn around. Another step or two, and I would have fallen to my death down a crevasse. Shaken, I returned to the settlement, glad to be alive and more appreciative of my wife, my family, and everyone else whom I had gotten to know at Grise.

Sam Willy was among the many who displayed a long-suffering patience when facing the harsh elements, disappointments, and unpredictability of living so far north. He showed great dignity and composure when dealing with embarrassing moments. One day, while carrying two steaming honey bags, one in each hand, down the school steps, he slipped and fell. Covered with human waste, which congealed and froze to his clothes, he took off for home, only to arrive back that afternoon as if nothing out of the ordinary had happened. Sam was the kind of man who, like many other Inuit, was underestimated and misjudged as innocent and somewhat primitive. To the contrary, he was as Arctic streetwise as any Inuit person from Resolute who had been saturated with the presence of outsiders wanting to make deals with the "Huskies" they met. I could just see Sam Willy not buying into anyone's game. I could see him pulling the sleeve of his parka up, displaying a fine watch, checking the time, turning his back, and walking away to get on with his affairs.

I respected Sam Willy and those in the community

like him. Here was a man of quiet dignity. One couldn't help but feel for him, though. Once, he—having looked forward practically all year for a mail order radio to come with the Christmas airdrop—was handed a crumbled package. It contained the shattered bits of his radio.

The airdrop event began with the dogs, which, outnumbering the people, howled in unison on hearing the sound of the Hercules aircraft, long before our ears detected it. Many gathered on the sea ice on that frigid, clear moonlit night waiting expectantly for the first parachute to appear. Then the chutes, carrying large baskets full of mail and Christmas gifts, came crashing down on the ice. There were cheers. Soon after, peering eyes saw the plane's blinking wing and tail lights fade away. Then the police radio crackled, and the pilot called out, "Tell us to clear the site. There is one more drop . . . Are you the schoolteacher?"

I replied, "No, I'm his wife."

He then said, "So you must be the Queen of Ellesmere Island."

I suppose it must have been Lesley's English accent. Then the deafening rumble of the Hercules echoed around the fjord again. It roared over and dropped, would you believe it, a real Christmas tree! Imagine, far above the tree line in the High Arctic, not many miles from the north pole, a Christmas tree. Soon after the drop, it became the centrepiece for Christmas celebrations in the schoolhouse.

There were many surprising items found a way into Grise Fiord. The local co-op, owned by the people but operated by the "policee," had a warehouse. In the warehouse, it was alleged one could even find a case or two of V-Master cigarette papers, but no machines to roll them with. What was missing in the store stock were Ski-Doos. Allegedly, the RCMP wisely didn't encourage the use in and beyond the settlement. Why? They didn't want the Grise Fiord hunters contributing to the depletion of the polar bear population. It was felt the polar bears wouldn't have much of a chance. Moreover, dogs could help a starving hunter survive. But a person couldn't eat a Ski-Doo, and if an engine broke down, the chances of survival were slim. However, it was different with dogs. Even if only one or two dogs survived, we could get the hunter home. Dogs could also detect thin ice. A Ski-Doo might drop through the ice without warning, taking the driver with it. It all sounded so reasonable. Yet what seemed the adoption of a "necessary" paternalistic attitude by the RCMP may not have sounded politically correct. I wondered how the Inuit felt.

No matter what decisions previous RCMP made, Lesley and I appreciated Lorne and Tom's generosity and thoughtfulness. They shared their fresh meat supply with us by having us over for meals. When their meat supply was low, or it became a little ripe, they doctored it up and still made us welcome at their table.

The Inuit families were also very generous in supplying us with seal liver, through trade from our rations, or as gifts. That was a real treat. Still, I tried to get some fresh meat shipped up myself from Frobisher. I asked the visiting administrator at the time to have some sent up when he got back to Frob. But true to his reputation of batting a low average when following up on requests, he didn't get me my meat. I should have known and taken seriously the joke that was going around. On taking off from a settlement, one would see torn pages from his notebook drifting down like wartime pamphlets. Again, I tried to order meat by radio. I received a case of yeast instead. Could it have been bad radio reception down in Frob, or . . . ?

Tom and Lorne, like many living in the north, appeared to develop rituals to avoid cabin fever. Most of us know that a person's little idiosyncrasies can, in time, become blown out of proportion, causing people to really get on each other's nerves. I believe that Tom and Lorne had their guarded allocated seat at their table. Tom kept his door shut during the night because he slept with his window open. Not Lorne! As the year progressed, I and I could also see us developing our ways of doing things to keep out of each other's hair. The dark times could have been devastating. But people visited. Children came and played with Andrew and Mark. Lesley and I would respond to some invitations to get out and about. Sometimes we would go for walks when the weather would allow it. We would set out on the sea ice to view the bead of buildings running along the shoreline. I would pull the boys in a heavy replica of a full-size komatik made by a kind Inuit fellow. Its runners had a frozen porridge surface, which, like the real ones, could be shod with steel in the spring.

I did have one komatik ride with Tom. He had carefully packed the grub box, and yet somehow, to our amazement, we had a taste of kerosene-soaked donuts. Tom and Lorne took pride in our baking. The new flavour in our repertoire was unintentional and caused a few chuckles.

Sometimes, though, Tom had to do things that weren't funny at all. Straddling a monster of a husky dog named Duke, he unceremoniously yanked Duke's chin up, pried his mouth open and filed away at Duke's teeth. Old Duke, with tongue hanging out, frozen blood on his chin, must have known that he'd been bad in having chewed his harness for the umpteenth time. He submitted to the ordeal with barely a growl or whimper. Now there was a loyal, forgiving dog and a practical master. Working with the dogs was risky. But even more so was the harvesting of white whales for dog food. Those creatures swam in waters close by the settlement, which became a shooting gallery. Hunters out in boats shot down and toward the shore. Those on the shore shot down toward the boats. It's a wonder that only the unfortunate whales got killed. The choice of dog and people food was limited mainly to seal and fish for humans and whale for dogs. Muskox hunting was seriously frowned upon, as was hunting polar bear for meat, especially the bear's liver, which was toxic, containing high levels of vitamin A.

The three brothers, Akeeago, Apeelapic, and Mosesee (the Anglican catechist), who had come from Pond Inlet to settle in Grise Fiord, had been brought up to hunt in the High Arctic. They, with the former Quebec Inuit, showed great survival skills in providing for theirs and needy families. They even had enough energy left to be very hospitable. Lesley and I felt we were guests in their home, the land about us. I enjoyed Japattee and Siglook, who, like the rest of their classmates, would screw up little noses to indicate "No," and raise eyebrows to say "Yes." I appreciated Larry, who spoke English, having been south for eye treatment. I suggested he should get his education for sure because he wouldn't be able to survive in the Arctic as a hunter. He fooled me. Years later, he is one of the few that I knew who stayed on in Grise Fiord and did well.

I admired those, whether Inuit or white, who did stay. They would need a certain sense of self sufficiency, but even more, an inner strength to maintain mental health, for the vast expanse of ice and snow, exaggerated by the intensity of light and dark, could make a person feel so insignificant. It is no wonder one gets a feeling of being a mere snowflake in a land where the Inuit people had many different words for snow.

Even when looking up into the sky, as Olaf and I did one day during the perpetual light, I felt for Lesley and our boys, who were very much deprived.

Thousands of feet up, a plane passed overhead. We could see its exhaust plume etched in the intense blue. Olaf remarked, "Yah, yah, just think, those people up there are sitting in their shirts and ties, with polished city shoes, smiling, drinking, and enjoying a comfortable warm plane going somewhere, and here we are."

Often, I would recite again the poem I had learned in grade school:

> "I see the lights of the village
> Gleam through the rain and the mist,
> And a feeling of sadness comes o'er me
> that my soul cannot resist" (Wordsworth 1807)

That sadness obviously manifested itself. For I would paint pictures that I later destroyed when I left Grise. Once, I even boiled a fox skull on the kitchen stove, cleaned and bleached it, and had it pose for one of those pictures. Thomas Hardy, the author of *The Return of the Native*, described the influence of the Egdon Heath on people. He put his finger on the fact that the environment we find ourselves in shapes our thinking. The High Arctic certainly influenced Lesley's and mine. I only wish today that I knew if and how it affected our two little boys in our short but intense stay in Grise Fiord. I sensed a need back then our need for assurance, Sometimes Mark would climb out of the high-walled crib a kind, local Inuit man made for him and crawl into our room and hoist himself onto our bed. Andrew would often appear in the doorway. He'd stand silently staring at us. We wondered if he was just making sure that we were still there.

Another person from the south, from northern Quebec, was also affected by the long, dark winters and perpetually light summers. Possibly through no fault of his own, the land drove him a little mad. As a result, he scared the life out of many residents, and intimidated others, for fear of what he might do. Though small in stature he reminded me of the villain dressed in black who faced Gary Cooper in *High Noon*. The hunters gathered with Tom and Lorne to work out a plan to keep this guy in check till we could ship him out. The men were afraid of leaving our women and children alone in Grise when we went hunting, for fear that he would stay behind and take advantage of us.

We knew of murders committed in the Arctic. I, too, had heard about us. The word was out that the judge of NWT collected Eskimo carvings depicting murder scenes. So that was on our minds when we left Grise, travelling south on the same plane as this man, who'd been banished from Grise. My fear faded though, when on a stopover in

Frobisher, one of our sons toddled over to him and

looked up at him. I think I saw a tear appear in the corner of his eye. Rather than threatening, that pathetic man looked so lonely and lost.

Had Lesley and I stayed longer, who knows how we would have appeared. Would we have had the mental stamina to confront the deep, dark winters and intensely light summers again? We would never find out. We were grateful that I got a transfer to Fort Chimo in northern Quebec, where, after several months, I won a competition to become an Arts and Crafts Development Officer.

Chapter 9: Self-Help Insights and Activities

When the onlooker was in his loud, pimply, awkward teens, he suffered from boils. His mother knew the cure contained powerful stuff that he'd rather not know about. All that he wanted to know was if it worked. Would it draw out the dregs, clearing the way for healing? It did.

The onlooker, reflecting deeply on what he absorbed through his senses while frequenting the park, recalled that experience. He saw the power of the park in its more spiritually elevating way, bringing forth from the depths of his being what needed attention for restoration. After all had begun to surface as memories, ideas, responses to nature around him, and his belief he was part of it, all affirmed him, and he resolved to continue frequent Spirit Lake Park. He devised a liturgy that would help him feel he belonged to something greater than himself. He could not remember where he got these particular "seven words to live by," but he would take the liberty of using them as a vehicle to enhance his liturgy in motion.

A Week's Worth of Words to Live By

Live, Love, Learn, Laugh, Give, Try, and Think. Anon

He would reflect and ponder over one word per day as he circled the park's lake. During his first week's liturgy walks thoughts and ideas surfaced and varied according to the use for each day.

*

LIVE: Sunday. The medical doctor, musician, and missionary Dr. Schweitzer once wrote that people Id "reverence for life." Exactly what does that mean? In Thornton Wilder's play, Our Town a woman dies, but is allowed to choose one day to live over again. She chooses her twelfth birthday. It was then she had savoured and enjoyed everything around her. "You cannot look at everything hard enough." To her mother, she said in desperation, "Let's really look at it another time." Looking around her, she also said, "Earth, you're too wonderful to realize." I discovers I missed a lot while living.

When Alberta's Indian Chief Crowfoot lay dying, he

delivered his message to his tribe: "A little while and Crowfoot will be gone from among you. What is life? It is as the flash of a firefly in the night. It is as the breath of a buffalo in the wintertime. It is a little shadow that runs across the grass and loses itself in the sunset."

In a book entitled *The Touch of the Earth*, the writer, Jean Hersey, suggests,

> "It's important not to have one's life all blocked out, not to have the days and weeks totally organized. It's essential to leave gaps and interlude spontaneous action. Why? Because it is often in those moments, when we open ourselves to new, unlimited opportunities brought into our lives by chance, that our life paths take our most interesting turnings. That doesn't mean not visiting our favourite haunts."

The famous cellist Pablo Casal, even at age ninety-three, knew the importance of taking time for himself. He said,

> "For the past eighty years, I have started each day this way. It's not a mechanical routine but something essential to my daily life. I go to the piano, I play preludes, and fugues of Bach's. It's a sort of discovery of the world in which I have the joy of belonging. It fills me with the awareness of the wonder of life, with a feeling of the incredible marvel of being human. The music is never the same, never! Each day it is

something new, fantastic, and unbelievable." Pablo Cascal n.d.

Live each moment of our lives while taking in our surroundings. I regret that I didn't do that when I attended university grad. school. When I graduated, I said to , my wife, "What wonderful surrounding we live in!" Her valid response was, "You've just noticed? You've had your nose buried in your books. No wonder." She was right. I, in my struggle to survive academically, had missed so much!

In our struggle to survive, just to get through the day, what do we miss?

*

LOVE: Monday. Why love? A wise physician once said, "I've practised medicine for thirty years. I've prescribed many things. But in the long run, I've learned the best medicine is love."

Someone asked him, "What if it doesn't work?"

His answer: "Double the dose."

Merely believing, as a person of faith, isn't enough. The word "credo" does not solve the puzzle unless we add the word "amo," I love. The quote in the Bible is "Love one another."

Eddie Cantor wrote, "Love isn't like a reservoir. You'll never drain it dry. It's much more like a natural spring. The longer and further it flows, the stronger and deeper and clearer it becomes."

The practice of loving is made up of consistent unselfish acts. The fact is, "Love isn't eternal, it is day to day, it brings home the bacon and fries. It wipes noses, It makes the bed."

Sometimes it's even tough love. We love when we engage in the messy stuff of life for others. We accept that when we love ourselves, we can love others, knowing that our Creator loves us.

*

LEARN: Tuesday. Live, Love, Learn. It's sad that some people are brought up to think learning is a duty. Watch a baby learn to walk. The child obviously finds it exciting. The child is simply doing what one is designed to do, as we also are designed to do. Yet still we may ask, "Why learn anyway?" The answer? We learn to be at peace with ourselves. We learn what effect we have on other people. We learn so that we will have minds open to new experiences.

John Lubbock, English parliamentarian once said, "There are three great questions in life we need answers to over and over: Is it right or wrong? Is it true or false? Is it beautiful or ugly?"

Also, to learn to know ourselves is to know where we fit into the world, to learn what little thing we can give it. To know what little thing we can give is to know how much it can give us. But that learning process takes effort.

Lastly, Remember, learning only takes place when there is a change in behaviour.

*

TRY: Wednesday. There's no sense thinking we are going to learn life's lessons if we are afraid to get our feet wet. During a water safety course, a swimming instructor got this note from a worried mother: *My daughter will not be going swimming in the pool until she learns to swim.*

We are not going to go far in our life's journey, whatever path we choose, unless we risk and are willing to face new challenges regardless of age or physical shape.

The actress Sophia Loren, among many others, said, "I see myself as very fortunate living now when age isn't that much of a factor."

So if you put on weight, find that you need glasses, get a little pain in your knee, notice a few brown liver spots on your hands, don't despair. There's a fountain of youth. It is in your mind, your talents, the creativity of people you love. When you learn to tap this source, you will have defeated age."

It seems true, though, that as persons see more and more years pass, some confront learning more and more, and some stay on the same spot and give up trying to sample another space.

*

LAUGH: Thursday. Accept a need to Live, Love, Learn, Try laughing. It's good for the health as a great exercise. How so? When you explode into laughter, your diaphragm descends deeply into your body, and your lungs expand.

That greatly increases the amount of oxygen taken in. As it expands sideways, the heart beats faster and harder. Circulation speeds up. Liver, stomach, pancreas, spleen, and gall bladder are stimulated. A human's entire circulation system is stimulated. All of which confirms what a wise person said two thousand years ago. "Laughter is a bodily exercise precious to your soul." Anon

*

GIVE: Friday. Live, Love, Learn, Try, Laugh, and Give.

Sometimes giving may simply be an act of kindness. Albert Schweitzer lived and taught in Strasbourg, Germany. One day he and some friends sat together eating. It came to the dessert. The waitress brought big cake to the table. Schweitzer counted the people around the table. There were nine. But he cut ten pieces. Ten pieces when there were only nine? "Yes," he explained, "One piece for the young lady who graciously served us."

*

THINK: Saturday. Let us Live, Love, Learn, Laugh, Try, Give, and Think.

Our lives can affect not only other people, but also nature's other creatures, and our sensitivity to nature in our lives can also profoundly affect us.

The onlooker's visits to the park continued, and his life was enriched by his liturgical walks and sensitivity to the gifts that nature offered. As G.K. Chesterton said, "An adventure is only an inconvenience rightly considered. An inconvenience is only an adventure wrongly considered."

Concepts to Contemplate

I constantly revisited and thought about how these concepts applied in living out my life, before grieving the loss of Lesley, and after, during my grieving.

1. "Life goes on regardless of adversity, so persevere, live life to the fullest" Anon
2. We have three ages: mental, physical, spiritual
3. Three Types of Anxiety 1. Death 2. Emptiness 3. Meaninglessness 4. Guilt
4. Hegel's Thesis, Antithesis, New Thesis
5. Well of meaning from top down: 1. Pleasure 2. Power 3. Love 4. Meaning 5. Dignity
6. In conversation with others, the importance of measuring impact and response
7. Live between pain and pleasure
8. Basic needs. Every person has a right to say with conviction:
   - I am safe (security)
   - I am free (new adventures)
   - I am heard (recognition)
   - I count for something (recognition)
9. Some people live from the inside out, others from the outside in (empathy for others).

10. We are part of everyone we meet. Descartes's philosophy: "I think therefore I am" versus "You cannot be yourself without others." Anon

11. "You are not one person, but three: The one you think you are; The one others think you are; The one you really are Anon

12. Seek humanity, humility, humour

13. Types of power: manipulative, competitive, creative, nutrient

14. In conflict, it can be helpful hearing the "Prayer of St. Francis": "O Divine Master, Grant that I may not so much seek to be consoled, as to console; To be understood, as to understand. To love as to be loved."

15. In one-to-one conversations, question who is speaking. Is it a parent, child, or adult talking? If each plays the role of the parent, what then? If, similarly, it is child-child, or adult-adult, what then?

16. Bible uses threaded throughout describe human predicaments: 1. Bondage 2. Wilderness 3. Pilgrimage 4. Living with unresolved questions 5. Response 6. Responsibility 7. Power 8. Freedom

17. Learning only takes place when there is a change of behaviour.

18. Religions promising security: restless activity,

eroticism, trivia, totalitarianism

19. Big questions: Where did I come from? Why am I here? Where am I going?
20. If life is to be exciting, I can't play it safe.
21. The flaw in western philosophy is dualism. If you have this, you must also have that versus wholistic.
22. Desirable, i.e. flexibility, resilience
23. To define anything, I need contrast, need both darkness and light, negative and positive
24. Pulled, stuck, or taking own initiative to go forward in life
25. Light is life, darkness is death
26. There are many crosses and resurrections before we take our last breath.

Self Study: "Know Thyself"

<u>Know your strengths and limitations</u>. Identify psychological baggage accumulated over years.

1. First list: "I am's"
2. Then put + or – beside each
3. Third: count pluses and minuses
4. Result? A positive or negative self-image

Projects:

- What changes would you like to make for myself? For others? For your Creator?
- Draw your lifeline: a graph showing "put downs", "drop offs", "successes" throughout life.

Activities:

- Round the likes of Spirit Lake, meeting and visiting with people along the way
- Do Priscilla's assignments
- Choose from the above list of concepts & delve deeper into the significance of each
- Pray, for example: The Prayer of St. Francis, or others including these thoughts:
    - "Neither look to past with regret nor to future with apprehension" Anon

      "God help me stand for the hard right against the easy wrong" Anon
- Reconnect with nature (ecosystem), self, and others
- Seek to find meaning and existential significance in this

Afterword

I believe that, when really hurting, we, as creatures, tend to crawl away and hide to lick our wounds, maybe even die—if not in body, then in mind, longing to retreat back into our mother's womb where one is safe and cozy, NOT POSSIBLE! So, what then?

Thrown off kilter, suffering grief's vertigo I sought a way to defeat nasty stressors defined as uncontrollable, unpredictable, and inescapable. Grieving the loss of Lesley, I found I could no longer control or predict dementia's death blow. I couldn't even escape from inevitable painful feelings of remorse. So, what to do escape, leave the battlefield, give in to the tendency to hide away hurt somewhere, somehow to avoid too much coming at me from all directions? I knew deep down of a better way to deny despair; I considered choosing to re re-engage with nature and others to get unstuck to find a life.

But with Lesley gone, the question still lingered. Should I retreat back into a cave like Plato, seeing reflections of light from the cave entrance shadowed on a wall. Thinking that's all there is to look forward to without Lesley? Or do I step out into the park with others, contemplate, suck up life's juices, meet Spinoza, hear Priscilla, and enjoy the ride?

Answer? I'll choose the latter. How about you?

Places Where I and Ken Lived Through Our Sixty Years of Marriage

Question: would this many moves have contributed to Lesley's dementia?

Winnipeg, Manitoba

God's Lake Narrows, Manitoba

Norway House, Manitoba

Grise Fiord (Ellesmere Island), NWT

Fort Chimo, Quebec

Frobisher Bay, NWT (Iqaluit)

Ottawa, Ontario

Yellowknife NWT

Merrickville, Ontario

Yellowknife, NWT

Vancouver, BC

Herchel, Saskatchewan

Saskatoon, Saskatchewan

Glenboro, Manitoba

Moose Jaw, Saskatchewan

Fort Smith, NWT

Winnipeg, Manitoba

Mission, British Columbia

Taber, Alberta

Claresholm, Alberta

Lethbridge, Alberta

Victoria, British Columbia

Related Readings

Alcott, Louisa May, *Beginning Again*

Bible, "Ecclesiastes, 3:15 "

Bible, "1 Corinthians 13

Bible, Philippians, 3:14

Byron, Lord, "When We Two Parted"

Casals, Pablo, 'The capacity to care is what gives life its
    deepest meaning"

Chaucer, Geoffrey, *CanterburyTales*

Chekhov, Anton, *Three Sisters*

Chesterton, GK, *Saint Francis of Assisi*

Cohen, Leonard, *Anus*

Crassweller, Ken *The Power of Goose Island Park*

Crassweller Ken, *Here Comes the Bus*

Crowfoot, Chief, "His Dying Speech"

Daka, Kenneth & Terry *Martin, Grieving Beyond Gender*

Defoe, Daniel, *Robinson Crusoe*

Descartes, René, "I think therefore I am"

Douglas, Lloyd C, *White Banners*

Einstein, Albert, "Out of My Later Years"

Emerson, Ralph Waldo, "Self Reliance"

Emerson, Ralph Waldo, "There is a crack in everything
    God has made" Essay iii 1841 Composation pg15

Baldwin, Faith, "Many Windows: Seasons of the Heart"

Dobinsky, Leon, "We Rise Again", 1985

Einstein, Albert, "Letters"

Frankl, Victor ,*Man's Search for Meaning*

Godden, Rumer, *The River*

Hemingway, Ernest , *For Whom the Bell Tolls*
    & Farewell to Arms

Kaiser, *Garry Feathered Life* 3, page 73

Kübler-Ross, Elisabeth, *On Death and Dying*

Lennon, John and Paul McCartney, *Let It Be*

Lewis, C.S., *Mere Christianity*

Longfellow, Henry Wordsworth, "Nature", 1878

Longfellow, Henry Wordsworth, "The Day Is Done"

Loren, Sophia, "Fountain of youth is in your mind"

MacDonald, Coleman, *Once Upon a Little Town*

Magritte, Rene, "The Lovers", 1928

Manley, James K, "Spirit of Gentleness"

Mead, Margaret , *Continuities in Cultural Evolution*

Miller, Arthur, *"Death of a Salesman"*

Munch, Edvard, "Death Bed Scene"

Plato, The Republic, Allegory of the Cave.

Rubin, Simon Shimshon, *Working With The Bereaved:*
    Multiple Lenses on Loss and Mourning

Russell, Bertrand, *"The Conquest of Happiness"*

Sharpe, R. Lee, "Princes and Kings"

Santayana, George, *The Poet's Testament*

Schweitzer, Dr., "Reverence for Life"

Shakespeare, William, "All the World a Stage,"
    As You Like It" act 2, Scene 7
Shakespeare, William, *Hamlet*
Steinbeck John *Travels With Charley*
Thieck, Bob & George D. Weisse, "What a Wonderful
    World "
Thomas, Dylan, "Do No Go Gentle Into that Good Night"
Thoreau, Henry David, *Walden*
Thoreau, Henry David "Most men live lives of
    quiet desperation"
Tooker, Georg, "The Subway"
Tournier, Paul, *Solitude*
Vander Post, Lauren, *The Seed and the Sower*
Walton, Isaac, *The Complete Angler*
Wilder, Thornton, *Our Town*
Williams, Tennessee, *Orpheus Descending*
Williams, Tennessee, *The Glass Menagerie*
Whittaker, Roger, "Last Farewell",
Withers, Bill, "Stand By Me"
Wordsworth, William, "Wisdom and Spirit of
    the Universe"

Works Cited - Bibliography

Wild Goose Chase Inc. Blog. "Managing Fall Bird
    Migration." October 26, 2020.

Baldwin, Faith. *The Lonely Man.* Thorndike Pr., 1964.

Bereavement, Christopher Hall MAPS Australian
    Centre for Grief &. "Recent Developments in
    Understanding grief & Bereavement." *in Psch. Dec,
    Issue,* 2011.

C.S.Lewis. *Mere Christianity.* Harper Collin, 1952.

Chekhov, Anton. *The Three Sisters.* Moscow, 1901.

Coleman, MacDonald. *Once Upon a Little Town.* Red Deer
    Alberta: Kingfish Press, 1979.

Colleagues, Niamb McNam. "Community Identity for
    Personal Well Being." *British Journal of Social
    Psychology,* Oct. May 2001.

Einstein, Albert. "Einstein Quotes on Spirituality." *Simple
    Quotes to Remember Judaism On Line,* n.d.

Goodreads. "Pablo Cascal." n.d.

Goodreads.com. "Albert Einstein Quotes." n.d.

Managing Fall Bird Migration. Wild Goose Chase Inc.,
    October 26, 2020.

Miller, Arthur. *Death of a Salesman.* Viking Press, 1949.

Sarton, Mary. *Journey of a Solitude.* W.W.Norton and Company, 1938.

Sitwell, Edith. *Poems and Quotes.* n.d.

Thoreau, Henry David. *Walden ,civil disobedience, quotations, writings 3rd Edition.* W,W,Norton N.Y., 2008.

Tounier, Dr.Paul. *Escape From Loneliness.* SCM Press, 1976.

Wilder, Thorton. *Our Town.* Coward McCann, 1938.

Williams, Tennessee. *Orpheus Descending.* Dramatic Play Services, 1958.

—. *Orpheus Descending.* Dramatic Play Services, 1958.

—. *The Glass Menagerie.* NY: Random House, 1945.

Wordsworth, William. *Poems In Two Volumes.* 1807.

About the Author

Ken Crassweller is a retired United Church of Canada minister and the author of six previous books: *The Overturned Canoe* (2004), *Let Ookpiks Fly* (2004), *Here Comes the Bus* (2004), *The Power of Goose Island Park* (2005), and *Tools for Clergy* (2006) with Trafford Publishing, and *Peetakvik* (2022) with FriesenPress.

He lived with his wife, Lesley, for sixty years. Together, they adopted three children, Andrew, Mark, and Marnie. After Lesley's death from dementia on November 20th, 2021, Ken began writing *Determined to Get a Life* as a way of making sense of his grief and finding closure.

Ken lives in Glenshiel Independent Living Facility in Victoria, B.C.

Printed in Canada